HOW TO RUSH SLOWLY . . .

AND AVOID PANIC ATTACKS

. . . A SELF-HELP THERAPY BOOK.

AGNES STEVEN

THE
LAID BACK
PRESS

First published in 1998 by
Cromwell Publishers, Manchester
Paperback ISBN 1 901679 30 6

This edition published in 1999 by
The Laid Back Press
15 Carrick Road, Ayr KA7 2RA, Scotland, UK
+44 (0)1292 283021

Typesetting and print production by
Gilmour Print, Stewarton, Ayrshire KA3 3EL
www.ictus.co.uk

Paperback ISBN 0 9536477 0 6

CONTENTS

Dedication

I dedicate this book to my husband Andy, who has travelled with me through the good years and the bad, and who has worked on his own personal development. I have never doubted his love for me.

Andy and I are eternal children and hopefully we can teach other people that fun and laughter is the ultimate healer. Regardless of what is wrong, no matter what has happened in your life, if you can learn to laugh again you have the best medicine available. It is possible to feel young, vibrant, healthy. You can feel that life is wonderful to wake up to in the morning. This is the philosophy of our lives and one that we hope to go on teaching people for as long as we are able.

I would like also to dedicate this book to my parents, my darling mother Kitty and my dear father William. I congratulate them on the wonderful job they did in bringing up myself, and my sisters and brother, Christina, Catherine and William. I thank my niece Catrina and my nephews Bobby and Calum for the fun they have given me over the years. I thank all my family for the time that I share with them all.

I wish to thank those in the medical profession for their support over the years.

I especially thank my own patients who have taught me much about life. I hope I have given as much to them as they have given me.

I would like to thank Elizabeth Blair who helped me in the writing of this book. She spent many hours with me and many more hours alone, deciphering every passage. She has given me time and patience and has the knack of putting into words exactly how I feel.

I am very lucky in life. My husband is my best friend. My partner in life. We have made the journey of self-discovery together and, like swans, we are paired for life. If our parents were alive today they would have been so proud of what we have achieved together.

I must also thank a very special friend who died just a few years ago. My cat TC was with me for fifteen years and taught me all there is to know about relaxation and about getting the most out of life. With his three and a half legs TC managed more than most of his four-legged compatriots.

Finally, I'm always telling people that they should give themselves a pat on the back for their achievements regardless of how trivial they may seem. (I've actually been nicknamed Agnes 'pat-yourself-on-the-back' Steven.) We just don't give ourselves enough praise. So, I'm going to end this dedication by giving myself my pat on the back for completing the book. I hope it gives you the help and encouragement you need.

From the Author:

On 20th February 1981 at 1.25pm precisely, I entered a living nightmare that was to dominate and control every aspect of my life for the next two years.

On that day, as on every other, I called to visit my mother. When there was no response to my repeated ringing of her doorbell I realised that something was terribly wrong. I tried to break down the door, and swear that for a short time I became insane. The terror I was feeling was so bad.

- I panicked.
- I choked.

My worst fears were realised when my mother was found dead, and from then on I began to lose control.

- I was afraid of choking (hysteria in the throat);
- I was afraid of open spaces with people in them (agoraphobia);
- I was afraid to attend social occasions (social phobia);
- I was deeply depressed and suicidal, even eating and drinking was difficult.

I was on the road to self-destruction.

Outwardly I must have appeared quite normal, but inside

my head I was living through hell.

'Why does everyone else look so happy and relaxed? What is this terrible thumping in my heart? It must be a heart attack. Yes, I have such a tightness in my chest. My stomach is churning, my fingers are tingling and my legs are like jelly. I am sure my head is going to explode. Am I really dead?' I didn't know. At that time everything and everyone seemed unreal.

Such thoughts were crippling my life and I remember screaming silently, inside myself: 'Help me, help me, someone please help me.'

But no-one heard.

'These headaches can't just be tension. I must have a brain tumour. These feelings of sickness in my stomach can't be nerves. I must have cancer. I can't even see properly. There are black dots floating in front of my eyes. Is God paying me back? Am I being punished? I must have done something terrible to be made to live through such purgatory and suffering.'

In my darkest moments I did think of suicide. I became angry at the thought of having to live because of my husband and family. They could live a normal life while I was programmed to self-destruct. No-one told me then that one day I would find a way out of this living hell. Fortunately, I had a wonderful doctor. He suggested **hypnotherapy**. I can never thank him enough.

And thus began my journey back to health. It was long and it was hard – the loneliest walk in the world. But I did it.

For the next two years I read everything I could find on the subject of 'nerves'. I desperately tried to help myself in any way I could.

As children we believe in a magic that makes good things happen. If only it were that easy. This book is not magic but it will help you on your journey, a companion on the road back to a normal life. It will serve as a reminder that you are not alone. It will help you to help yourself, to take control of your own recovery.

If I'd had a book like this when I was nervously ill, it would certainly have hastened my recovery and spared me much suffering. When I was nervously ill such a book didn't exist.

Which is why I've written this one.

Agnes Steven, 1995

About This Book

It is normal to be tense and anxious when faced with a stressful situation. Tension only becomes a problem when you experience it continually in your daily life and it is brought about by normal, everyday, ordinary situations.

If you live life feeling as though you've forgotten to remove the coat-hanger from your coat before you put it on, or if your face aches, your teeth are sore, your chest feels tight, your back aches and your legs feel like they have a ton of bricks attached, then you undoubtedly suffer from stress.

Sometimes learning to relax is all that is needed. Section II of this book will teach you relaxation exercises and how to use them. Practise these exercises daily until you can use them with ease. Then you will begin to see your symptoms improve until gradually the tension is gone. Keep practising and using the exercises whenever you find yourself in a stressful situation. Only then can you prevent the build up of tension from becoming a problem again.

This part of the book is for everyone. Read it, learn it, use it and keep it by you at all times for this is the way forward, the outlook to a happier, healthier, stress-free life.

For some people however, those symptoms are made

worse by certain situations. These are the people whose lives have become a minefield of anxiety and fear. For them the problem is much more acute and it may help for them to understand, not only what is happening to them physically, but to understand what may have caused the onset of their problems and to acknowledge what it can do to their everyday lives and to the people they know and love. Section I is dedicated to them.

Introduction

Without exception, we all have problems in our lives- even those among us who are apparently very happy, very relaxed and outwardly very confident.

But some people never seem to have any worries at all – does it simply mean that their problems aren't as great or as meaningful as ours?

Possibly, but highly unlikely.

So how do these people live their lives apparently without a care in the world?

Perhaps our problems aren't caused by people, or places, or circumstances, as we tend to think they are. Perhaps it's the way we react to these people, or places, or circumstances, that causes us the problem.

When we are anxious, when we get those gut feelings, those horrible, frightening, angry feelings, we blame the person or the situation for causing them. But consider for a moment the possibility that it is our reaction, our mental and physical turmoil that causes us so much distress. We are giving ourselves the problem. In other words, a problem's not really a problem until we decide to make it a problem.

Instead of being pro-active towards resolving the situation

we become very reactive towards our own feelings and to the symptoms of anxiety. We become emotionally crippled.

If we were to channel all our energies into resolving the situation there wouldn't be a problem, but all our energy is used up in our anxiety. Our bodies react by activating our inner panic button.

This is a physiological process that protected our primitive ancestors from danger by preparing their bodies to fight, run or otherwise react to an alarming situation. In today's world there is normally less risk from life-threatening situations but our physiology still ensures that we can prepare to defend ourselves in one way or another.

When something alarms us, our bodies react automatically and all our inner resources are channelled towards dealing with the situation. Heart beat, respiration, blood pressure and adrenalin production are all stimulated by the sense of danger. When the part of our mind that controls reason tells us there is no real danger to life or limb, it tries to suppress this physiological reaction. When suppression of the alarm mechanism fails, when all rational thought is overtaken by an overwhelming physical and mental reaction, all our energies are channelled into internal conflict.

The result is physical and mental confusion and a

realisation that we may be losing control.

If this sounds unbearably familiar then no doubt you suffer from over-anxiety and panic attacks – the inevitable result of an alarm mechanism that is out of balance. Panic attacks result from the undue anxiety which we suffer when our body reacts automatically to a situation which our conscious, rational mind cannot acknowledge as a legitimate threat, e.g., going into a crowded supermarket, getting on a bus, going outside.

The circumstances which caused that first spell of anxiety may never actually be repeated but, because our memories are particularly good at storing the details of a distressing incident, we are acutely aware of that initial experience and we learn to fear those circumstances. Once we have suffered our first panic attack we are afraid of having another. We now expect to feel the panic and so, when confronted again by similar circumstances, our anxiety spirals into another debilitating panic attack *'it's all happening again'*.

We learn to feel the fear and the loss of control because we expect it to happen.

Then when faced with the 'fight or flight' alternative we take the easy option. Or so we think. Running away from a situation gives an immediate, 'right there and then' reward. No more of the unpleasant feelings. In the long term however you're simply training yourself into a habit, the habit of always reacting to the feelings, the habit of avoiding any situation which triggers the fear. At first this seems to be the answer.

- Just avoid it.
- No problem.
- What a relief!

In fact, as you withdraw from these situations by staying indoors, by not travelling on the bus, by having someone else do the shopping, by avoiding meetings at work, then the fear begins to rule your daily routine and slowly, but surely, this fear becomes the most powerful influence on your life.

The power of the anxiety that shrinks your world reaches out and touches everyone around you, everyone close to you. It affects your partner, your children, your friends, your colleagues. You feel guilty and inadequate because you know your behaviour is irrational. You feel helpless and out of control. Communication with other people becomes more and more difficult. Life becomes more restricted. Your world gets smaller and smaller.

Gradually you learn to live like this.

Learning by association is a very normal human process. That's why simple anxiety can very quickly spiral into debilitating panic attacks. Nevertheless, anxiety and panic does not have to be totally incapacitating to have a profound and disturbing effect on your life. You may be 'coping' on a day to day basis but the strain of anticipation, of waiting for the terror to strike, can be immense.

Your life should not, and need not, be lived like this. The whole process of anxiety – fear – panic is reversible. As we have learned to feel anxiety and distress so we can re-learn our responses to the same situation.

This is partly based on understanding. Until you can fully understand the reason for your panic and the causes of your distressing physical symptoms you will continue to be at the mercy of your anxieties. A large part of your anxiety lies in not understanding what is happening to your mind and to your body. When you begin to understand you will learn how to eliminate fear from your life.

Chapter 1: Physical and Mental Well-being

1.1 The Physical State of Anxiety

Anxiety is something we've all experienced. It's uncomfortable for all, but for some people the extreme physical reaction they experience is so severe they think they are becoming seriously ill (as I did). Unpleasant symptoms such as tense muscles, trembling limbs, stomach upsets, headaches, difficulty in breathing or swallowing, are so disturbing as to frighten people into changing the way they live and limit the things that they do.

Most of these symptoms are actually due to increased muscle tension. Perhaps the most common example is the tension headache. Increased tension in the muscles of the neck puts pressure on the scalp causing severe pain and a feeling of pressure in the head. The most important thing to remember is that although these symptoms may not be caused by actual physical illness they are, nevertheless, very real. They are not 'all in the mind'. The pain, sweating, trembling, and breathing problems are not in your imagination. They are caused by your nervous system over-reacting to a situation which you find stressful. If these symptoms appear suddenly they can cause you to panic. It is often difficult to work out why the symptoms have developed and it is not always necessary to know why. Worrying about it will only increase your state of anxiety and make the symptoms worse. It is better to look forward and try to make yourself feel better than to worry about why it started in the first place.

People are not always aware that physical and mental well-being are so closely related, or, that psychological problems can trigger the mechanisms in our body which cause us to feel unwell. Conversely, if you are not physically fit and well, you may be more prone to attack by psychological problems.

One of the most publicised and widely acknowledged contributors to good physical health is diet. Eating a well-balanced diet is vital for maintaining good health and energy levels. The most important, and yet most neglected, meal of the day is breakfast. Eat a good breakfast which includes protein (meat, fish, eggs, pulses, cheese, nuts, milk) and you won't experience that mid-morning energy drop which is caused by low blood sugar. When blood sugar levels are low you experience that familiar craving for sweet things. But beware, eating these can give what is known as a false lift – a sudden burst of energy and then an equally sudden drop leaving you feeling 'low'. Despite the expression 'low blood sugar', sugar is not what your body requires. It requires protein found in cheese, milk, meat, eggs, nuts, pulses etc. These foods release the right chemicals in a slow, controlled manner into the bloodstream helping maintain energy over a longer period of time and preventing your body reacting like a yo-yo. The craving for sweet things that you have may be confusing but substitute the sweet food with protein and you should notice the difference.

Another important aspect of our lifestyle which affects our physical health is sleep. Not sleeping, or insomnia is often associated with stress and usually it is worry and tension which keeps us awake at night. But, if you eat a large meal late in the evening your digestive system will be forced to work overnight. This may prevent your body mechanisms from slowing down and prevent you from having a good night's sleep. Similarly tea, coffee or other stimulants should be avoided at night. If you are suffering from stress your body needs all the help it can get, so look after it, no one else will.

1.2 The Physical Symptoms and What Causes Them

While you may be experiencing a whole range of frightening physical symptoms it would be wrong to assume that this is the actual problem. If you are very anxious your problem will be much more complex and the only way forward is to treat the anxiety. This will in turn alleviate your physical symptoms. Treating the physical symptoms will not cure your anxiety state. However, if you begin to acknowledge and understand these physical symptoms they will become less frightening and less worrying and hence will not add to your anxiety. Knowing that your body and not your mind is responsible will help you come to terms with your symptoms.

Headaches

From time to time everyone experiences tension headaches which are caused by a tightening of muscles in the back of the neck. When this happens your scalp becomes tight and you feel pressure on your head often behind your eyes. The muscles in your neck will be sore to the touch. Massage, and relaxation exercises will sometimes help to relax the muscles.

Palpitations

That alarming feeling you get when your heart races and beats very fast or when it seems to 'stop' suddenly and miss a beat is your heart reacting to the adrenalin produced when you become tense and anxious. These changes in the beat of your heart are called palpitations. There is nothing wrong with your heart but these feelings can be very distressing and may cause you to panic which of course produces more adrenalin and makes the situation worse.

Breathlessness

Sometimes your chest may feel tight and small, there's no room for your lungs to expand and you can't get a good deep breath. As a result you feel breathless and panicky, fearful that you might not be able to breathe at all. This feeling comes on when you become anxious and the chest muscles become tense. It will not prevent you from breathing.

Swallowing difficulties

Stress and anxiety cause your body to react by drying up your saliva. As a result you have to keep swallowing to clear your mouth, the muscles in your gullet tighten up and you feel as though you will choke. Often you will feel sick. If you are the type of person who is anxious in company then eating with other people can become a nightmare. Your gullet becomes so tight that the food will not go down and you feel that you can't swallow. You feel like you have a lump in your throat.

Aches and pains

Many people who suffer anxiety and stress experience pain, often in the chest – a cramping feeling that causes many people to believe they are suffering a heart attack. If your problems are not associated with your heart (and only your doctor can give you this reassurance) it is probably a direct result of your anxiety state. The excess adrenalin produced when you are anxious causes muscles to contract or go into spasm. When this happens to the muscles on the chest wall the pains that result can be so severe as to make you feel that you must be seriously ill.

Tiredness

Although you may go to bed early and sleep all night, your muscles will be so tense that you will not feel well rested. Your muscles start the day tense and stay that way and you feel constantly tired.

1.3 Fear and Panic

What you experience during any of these symptoms is an over-reactive nervous system. Adrenalin which stimulates your body to cope in difficult situations is over-produced. As a result your body over-reacts by producing physical symptoms. Your symptoms are very real. They are physical symptoms. They are not in your mind. But, because these symptoms worry and distress us we learn to anticipate them and to worry about them happening again. 'Will it be today?, Will it happen now?, Will I make a fool of myself?' It is fear of the symptoms which is disabling. It is the fear which causes us harm, which rules our life and which in turn makes us more nervous, more anxious and ultimately more tense. The fear becomes the problem.

When we have suffered the onset of some or all of these symptoms we begin to worry – 'Why did it happen?, When will it happen again?' We feel afraid. The fear makes us more anxious. When we find ourselves in a stressful situation we may suffer a sudden attack where powerful symptoms can hit us very quickly. Your heart begins to race, you feel weak, dizzy, breathless. This feels like an emergency. You panic. You are terrified. Afterwards you will feel completely normal but you begin to wonder...why? Next time you find yourself in a similar situation your body cues the release of adrenalin and off you go again. The vicious circle of anxiety, panic, anxiety has begun.

These symptoms are familiar to all anxiety sufferers. They are very distressing and very uncomfortable but the important thing to remember is that they can do you no actual physical harm. They are the physical evidence of a much more complicated and less recognisable problem. Understanding the nature and underlying cause of these symptoms won't make them go away but it does take away some of the mystery surrounding them, it allows you to stop worrying about them and it frees your mind to concentrate on addressing the real problems of tension and anxiety.

Chapter 2: Understanding Anxiety

Being tense means that your muscles tighten up, then the muscles around those muscles tighten up to protect them. This creates a situation called double tension and is the root of all your problems. Dealing with this tension is the basis for complete recovery. Addressing the physical symptoms and understanding how, and why, your body reacts to this tension is the first stage in the recovery process.

2.1 Phobias and Panic Attacks

If your life is ruled by fear and you spend all, or part, of your day being tense and anxious, fretting and worrying about the least little thing, then you are what is called an anxiety sufferer. If you have begun to avoid stressful situations that make you feel tense and anxious then you may have developed a phobia.

A phobia is sometimes called an irrational fear because it means you are frightened of something which is of no real physical danger to you. People can develop a phobia about almost anything: bees, being sick, going out, business meetings, buses, going bald, thunder, going to bed, injections, going blind... the list is endless. No matter how trivial or bizarre it may seem to others, a phobia causes real and terrible suffering, controlling lives and ruining relationships.

Agoraphobia is probably one of the most well known phobias and possibly one of the most debilitating. It is literally 'a fear of the market place' and is a fear of being in shops or buses, of visiting people, of being in open spaces or in busy public places. Half a million people in Britain are known sufferers at the present time. Two out of three sufferers are women. More women than men develop this particular phobia simply because their lifestyle leaves them more susceptible.

If you wake each morning with a terrible feeling of dread and gloom, wondering how you're going to face the day – how you're going to manage the shopping without panicking, or stand still in the bus queue or even hang out the washing, then you may be suffering from agoraphobia. You would rather go out in the dark when no-one can see you because you know that people are looking at you.

If perhaps you cannot bear the thought of being alone in the house, and you can't wait for the family to return home in the evening to rid you of your unpleasant thoughts and feelings then you may have a phobia called monophobia.

If meeting with, and talking to people fills you with dread, leaving you tongue-tied and panicky then you probably have a social phobia.

Most people today have heard something of anorexia, bulimia and compulsive eating disorder. These are all forms of eating phobia. You may feel you are always fat no matter how much or how little you weigh. You may eat and then vomit, binge and feel guilty, and tell yourself what a horrible person you are, how weak willed you are, and how only thin people are successful in this world.

No matter what kind of phobia you have, the stress and anxiety caused by the fear you are feeling causes the onset of a panic attack. It is the avoidance of situations in which you might panic that builds up a phobia in the first place.

2.2 Avoidance

However unpleasant it may feel, a panic attack will do you no physical or mental harm.

You may, however, experience one or more of the following symptoms: weakness, dizziness, choking, a feeling that you can't swallow or breathe correctly, tightness in your chest, jelly legs, pounding head, churning stomach, feeling sick, rapid heartbeat, feelings of unreality (knowing you are there but feeling that you are not).

You may feel that you are having a heart attack. If you are in any doubt about the source of your symptoms consult your doctor. You may find it hard to accept that nerves can give you all of these physical symptoms. If you have a sore throat, you know that it can affect your nose and ears. This is expected, but to accept that nerves can affect so many different parts of your body is hard.

Because a panic attack is so terrifying, as soon as you've had even just one you begin to avoid situations which may lead you to have another. The particular phobia which affects you will depend on which situations you are avoiding because of the panic attacks. The more situations you avoid, the more serious your phobia becomes and the more restricted your life will be.

In most cases the occurrence of an anxiety state is triggered by a long period of stress or a traumatic experience such as death, divorce, birth, marriage, change of job, retirement, redundancy or illness. The nervous system is at a low ebb and you are more likely to develop problems of this kind. Why it happens to one person and not another in the same circumstances is as yet unknown, though background and upbringing may be contributory factors.

You may begin to feel tense and anxious for some known and reasonable reason. You then begin to associate these unpleasant feelings with the normal places and situations in which you have been experiencing them. For example, if you are constantly worrying about your financial situation whilst shopping, then eventually you will begin to associate this worrying or anxiety, and its physical symptoms, with shopping. Just as certain places can hold happy associations you can develop anxious or unpleasant associations with places or situations. You then begin to expect these unpleasant feelings to occur and start to avoid these situations because doing so takes away the unpleasant feelings.

Every avoidance builds up the phobia, since each avoidance makes the next attempt even more difficult. That's why each person's phobia is unique to them – it depends entirely on the kind of situation they have been avoiding.

You may feel that your problem just struck out of the blue. But this is unlikely. The problem will have developed over a period of time without your having noticed it. Simply by association, your body has learned to react in a certain unpleasant manner to particular situations.

Just as you can learn desirable things such as reading or riding a bicycle, you can learn undesirable things. Reacting to normal situations with anxiety or a panic attack is simply an undesirable piece of behaviour which you have learned. You could call it a bad habit. What you must do now is learn to react normally to normal situations.

2.3 Controlling the Symptoms

Breathing is an activity we take for granted. Few of us realise, until it becomes a problem, that breathing is a technique that can be controlled, and improved upon, and used in our everyday lives to control our physical and mental well-being.

When you are tense and begin to feel panicky, your heart speeds up, your breathing speeds up and your heart speeds up some more, sending blood racing around your body. The physiological effect of this is to set the adrenal glands going. The tiny adrenal glands sit just above your kidneys and are controlled by your nervous system. They secrete a very powerful hormone called adrenalin when we respond to a stress situation. Adrenalin affects the working of all your major organs and hence can cause some very powerful reactions! Adrenalin floods in to your body causing the horrible feelings you associate with a panic attack – thumping heart, jelly legs, altered vision, upset stomach. I always used to imagine it like a fizz in my blood. As the heart thumps faster, all the symptoms like dizziness and unreality return. This is why relaxation is so important to your recovery. The secret of proper relaxation, physical or psychological, is to slow down the heart rate and take control of your breathing.

The relaxation techniques described in Section II will help you slow down your heart rate. By slowing down your heart the blood won't race through your body and this means the adrenal glands don't release the chemicals that cause the terrible feelings.

There is in fact, no physiological difference between feeling frightened and feeling excited. One of the amazing things about these glands is that they respond in exactly the same way to both situations. The chemical reaction within your body is exactly the same, so the basic reaction to fear and to pleasure is the same. It is how we interpret the feelings that makes the difference. It is how you deal with them that matters.

Just imagining your next panic attack can give you the symptoms. The only way to control these feelings is to learn to control your breathing, to slow it down. As we relax, our breathing becomes slower, deeper, more controlled.

Concentrate on breathing out. As you breathe in your muscles lift and tighten. When you breathe out your muscles relax and let go.

Take it one step at a time. Imagine that as you slowly breathe in, your heart beat will slow down, not immediately, but in a short time, and as you slowly breathe back out, it continues to slow.

Stick at it. Refuse to give in. It is important to practise relaxation or self-hypnosis at least once every day. I assure you that these methods work. Breathe slowly and your heartbeat will begin to slow down. Your blood will stop racing around your body. Everything will seem to slow down.

If it helps, imagine I am with you, talking to you and encouraging you. Remember that I know how you feel. I have been there. As you begin the lonely walk to recovery take comfort in the knowledge that I am there with you, your friend, helping and encouraging you along the way.

2.4 Controlling the Fear

Not surprisingly, most people expect to have recovered when the panic attacks stop happening. Not so. Recovery is knowing you have control, knowing that you can accept all these strange feelings you experience. If you never had another panic attack how would you know if you could deal with it if it did happen? You wouldn't know, and your life would be spent wondering. You would live in fear of the possibility of an attack and how you would control it if it happened.

The real cure is knowing you are in control when you feel the first signs of a panic attack starting. You need to know that if they come back you can take charge. The panic attack is no longer controlling you.

Learning to control your breathing is the key to taking control of your life. Learn to relax, learn to breathe. Concentrate on breathing out, control your heart rate and slow it down. Everything else will follow.

When you first start on the relaxation exercises you may be surprised at how you feel as you begin to relax. You may be frightened by what you feel. You might become panicky about feeling good and tighten up again. It's a vicious trend which we must slow down and reverse. We are dealing with double tension and double fear. We are afraid of the fearful feelings and fearful thoughts. It takes time to trust yourself, to acknowledge that it's O.K. to feel relaxed.

When we learn to relax and enjoy the natural feeling, we learn to take chances with our life. If we don't take these chances, we stay locked in the darkness – and it is indeed a total darkness. No-one, unless they have been there, can possibly understand how you feel. There is nothing outwardly visible to let people know how much you are suffering. If you tell people you feel frightened, terrified even, but you don't know what it is that is frightening you they assume you're stupid, neurotic...or just plain crazy! How can you not know what it is that frightens you? But you are afraid of the fear. It's fear upon fear.

The relaxation and self-hypnosis techniques help you take control of that fear. As well as making you feel relaxed, they help you turn that fear to anger.

Refuse to live your life like this! Don't let the fear rule your life!

Talk to yourself as to an imaginary person or to an enemy. 'You will no longer make me live like this. I refuse to live like this any longer.' Use the anger positively.

2.5 Controlling Your Life

Because of the fear and the tension your world has been restricted, becoming so small and so locked in on yourself that you feel this is your form of security. But your security soon becomes your insecurity when you have eventually locked yourself in so far that you can't step over your front doorstep, you are afraid to get on the train to go to work, afraid to go on the bus, afraid to drive your car, or you are afraid to go in to meetings because you know within yourself that you are going to feel those feelings. You think things before you can physically feel them. Although you may not be fully aware psychologically of the thoughts, at the back of your mind is the question 'what if...?' What if..., becomes a part of everyday life. 'What if the feeling comes back?' is your biggest fear. Then, because you think it, your body responds and you begin to feel it. What the mind thinks, the body follows through.

Whatever technique you choose to help you relax, if you stick at it and practise every day you will soon begin to realise that you can change the 'what ifs...', and your body will soon get used to the feelings of relaxation. At the moment, your body is so used to being tense that when you begin to relax, it will immediately tighten up again in response to these 'unusual' feelings. You have become so used to having the tension it has become a part of your life and you have learned to live with it. You must turn this tension into positive tension and positive stress.

When you begin to relax, your mind will pick up on the feelings of relaxation. Your body likes it and your mind likes it. Then you will become more aware of tension creeping back into your life and you are now in a position to deal with it before it takes hold again. Until now tension has been the norm, and it will take you some time to learn to live without it.

So, take it one step at a time. You may feel that you take one step forward, then two steps forward and one step back, but you have started to give yourself choices again. Your world is getting bigger and bigger.

Only you can take control of the suffering. You are the only person with the power to turn things around and give yourself a better life.

You can't expect anyone else to do it for you. You must commit yourself to doing relaxation exercises daily, and you must persist in trying tapes and techniques until you find one that works for you.

The hardest thing about getting better is the fear of being happy. You are too frightened to be relaxed because it is so long since you felt those happy feelings. You fear something will happen to spoil things if you dare to feel them again. You feel that something happened to get you like this in the first place. You feel that you are going to be disappointed again. You fear something happening and you are afraid that you won't be able to cope if it does. You feel that you will be paid back for being happy, or for being too smart.

This is not true.

Realise that what is going to happen will happen anyway. It's how you deal with it that counts. When you stay in your safe little world you think negative things won't happen to you. When you shut yourself away, your life becomes smaller and smaller and you think you can be safe. You feel that the world out there is a threat. It's not that you can't handle a situation, it's simply that you can't handle the feelings you have in that particular situation. Next time you have a panic attack, ask yourself what it is that really worries you, what it is that really angers you. You will find there is always a reason. Confront that reason and take control of your life.

Chapter 3: Understanding Ourselves

The basis of our personality, our self esteem, is formed in childhood. By the age of three we have discovered who we are. We already have thoughts about ourselves and we have learned more than a few of our characteristic traits and habits – good and bad!

3.1 Rejection

When we are children we look to the adults in our life for guidance on how to behave. We learn to react to the adults around us. On some days our childish pranks and mischief are tolerated or perhaps even treated with affection. On a different day, however, we may be chastised by the same adult for doing exactly the same thing. Through the inconsistencies of adult behaviour we learn to feel guilt, to accept the judgement of others and to assume the labels given us by other people. From being a child who is by nature happy, at ease and at peace with himself we begin to feel that we must be a bad person. What we don't realise, in our childish naivety, is that the person who really has the problem is the adult who is bringing his own fears and insecurities into our lives.

When similar situations arise, the child begins to experience negative emotions, a 'gripping' feeling inside, without understanding why. Now he feels the need to seek approval when he next comes into contact with that adult (who may well be a parent) because, naturally, he doesn't like the feelings of rejection he experienced last time. He doesn't want to be seen as a 'bad' person again. Suddenly, from being a relaxed and emotionally secure child he starts to feel uptight. Worse, the feelings are such that when he is enjoying himself he feels that something bad will happen to him, that he'll get into trouble. The child now becomes nervous, frightened of being happy, frightened of feeling secure, frightened of taking chances. He begins to doubt the feelings of security he once had. By now insecurity has probably started to creep into his life.

It soon starts to spread into other areas.

At pre-school and primary school we learn to cope with different situations and to interact on a daily basis with other adults – teachers, who inadvertently bring their own agenda and personal problems and insecurities into our lives. Teachers will often claim that a child is not concentrating or is easily bored. He finds it difficult to maintain the child's interest and blames the child. What many teachers don't recognise is that when a child's mind 'wanders' into fantasy it is, in effect, self-hypnosis which should be encouraged and used by the school to help develop the child's mind. But teachers, like all adults, bring their own problems in life to work. No matter how hard we try, it is very difficult to separate all the different parts of our lives. We look to vent all our pent-up emotions in the easiest way we can, we take the line of least resistance, the route that will have fewer repercussions. We, as adults, will take out our frustrations on the sensitive child. The child who is strong enough to answer back is not the child we choose to pick on. Sensitive children begin to seek approval in school, continually asking if everything is alright, are they doing well enough in class? This need for approval from teachers spreads to other adults, to parents, to neighbours. They may feel that their friends are better than they are.

The loss of self esteem has begun.

With the teenage years and secondary school comes the dreaded exams. Children can become terrified, always feeling the need to succeed and fearing failure. But is it really fear of failure we feel at this stage or is it fear of success? After all, if we succeed everyone expects us to succeed from now on. How well we do is pointed out to us, but failure is not always treated with the compassion we need and deserve. Generally we are not told that 'it doesn't matter' or 'never mind you'll do better next time'. The need to compare ourselves with others, with friends, with classmates has arisen. Competition has entered our life and with it the feeling of always having to try harder.

Primary school does afford some degree of security in our lives in that we see the same faces of classmates and teachers daily over a long period of time. With secondary school, however, not only have we lost that particular element of security but we now have to deal with puberty and with the social element of 'growing up', learning to interact with others. We are now expected to deal with things in a different way. But where do we actually learn to feel comfortable and confident within ourselves and with other people? These skills are not taught in school. Combine this with puberty and an adolescent interest in the opposite sex and we inevitably become mixed-up and confused young adults.

Much of how we react to these changes taking place in our life depends on our background and upbringing. Those who have a happy and stable home life are most likely to weather the storm and emerge as mature, capable and confident adults. Sadly there are many who do not. There are children for whom alcohol or an unhappy marriage has a huge impact on their life and long term frame of mind. There may be several children and an exhausted mother who is trying to run her life, be housewife, and mother, and hold down a job. There just isn't enough time or energy to spend on each child individually. Again there is the element of competition as each child vies for parental attention. An only child will fare little better. In their life pressure comes from parents who pin all their hopes and unfulfilled ambition on the child. Parents feel they are judged by the performance of their children but the responsibility to do better and to try harder lies with the child.

As teenagers we go through the rebellious phase as we try to make our mark on life, developing our own self and saying what we feel. This often is manifest in the way we dress and by our actions. Those of us who have been 'model' children suddenly break out. No-one is going to tell us what to do ever again. Parents become confused. As children we are even more confused because our minds are so easily influenced at this stage in our development.

There may be someone in our peer group who appears very relaxed and at ease with himself. But we can't see what is in their mind, we don't know what is going on in their head. We can only guess. We try to imagine that we do know and we start trying to become like this person, modelling our life on theirs, acting out their life thinking that this will make us happy – trying to be someone else because we are so unhappy with our own lot in life. It only makes us more unhappy because we don't get the fulfilment, we don't get the feelings we think we should get. Instead we feel guilt because we know we're upsetting our parents, we know our school work is suffering. Thoughts of the future disappear because our only thought is that we want to be free. We want to go out and be the real person who is inside us. But we don't know who that person is because that real person has only begun to develop.

Before we really have time to develop and become our own person we leave school and our friends and go out into working life. When we're at school there is still another person to take overall responsibility for our life. We can always get a note to explain why we've been absent or to excuse us from certain things. When we go out to the big wide world we must start dealing with different situations every day. We can't get a 'sick' note any more. We are faced with responsibilities we've never had to accept until now, responsibilities we don't know how to deal with and that we can't avoid.

It may be, that in our rush to join the adult world, we jumped into a job that was available at the time but wasn't really what we wanted. Before long we stop looking forward to work. Inside we begin to feel angry and resentful. Then we want things to make us feel better. This is when alcohol starts to play a part in our life. Instead of going out with friends and really enjoying ourselves we think that alcohol will help make us feel happy. But when we are out with friends and see them enjoying themselves we think that it is not happening for us. After a few drinks all the feelings of unease begin to surface. Drinking becomes uncomfortable because at the end of the night we are in tears knowing that we feel unhappy but not knowing what to do about it. We feel that others don't want to socialise with us any more. Some people may be unkind enough to tell us in the wrong way why they won't go out with us any more. Others may take us aside and explain more kindly. But it isn't easy to understand. All you feel is the rejection.

At this stage self esteem is so low that it will help enormously to have someone to talk to about your feelings. If there is no help available at this stage, life continues down the same path. You may feel that the thing you need to make life interesting is to get married and have children or to have children without the marriage. However, you still feel unhappy inside. You feel that you don't have this secret confidence you imagine everyone else has. You may then begin to suffer panic attacks. Frightened to go out. 'Why is it that everyone else feels so happy.' 'Why is it that everyone else is so much in control.'

3.2 Counselling

Everything we feel starts from way, way back. Everything we are as an adult is a legacy from our childhood. People sometimes say that it doesn't matter where our problems have come from – deal with them now. Sometimes, however, we have to go back, to look and to see where these problems started. We could all say that we've had problems in our childhood, everyone has. We can't keep using them as an excuse for things that go wrong in our life. We must do something to stop the downward spiral. If problems do come from childhood it is very helpful to see someone who is not only a counsellor but who will carry out analysis. During analysis you can be taken into hypnosis and regressed back to anything in your past that may be causing you problems now. Feelings are stronger than any of our conscious thoughts and emotions. If you keep having feelings of unhappiness but don't know why, or maybe you do know why but don't know what to do about it, then you may need to see a counsellor who is also a psychoanalyst and hypnotherapist.

To find a reputable counsellor or psychoanalyst ask your GP to recommend one or ask around for other people's experiences. Find out what qualifications any practising analyst or counsellor has before agreeing to a consultation. Ask for a recommendation from the professional association. There are many horror stories about unqualified and disreputable practitioners in this field and you should always double check. Hopefully, before too long, there will be a professional register of analysts and counsellors who have reached a minimum standard of qualifications and experience before being allowed to practice. One of the best qualifications your counsellor/therapist can have is that they have been there themselves. Then you won't feel judged by them and you are more likely to identify with each other. Don't be afraid to ask if they have any personal experience of life's problems before making an appointment.

Some people go through most of their life before realising their self esteem is so low. Should you, at this point in the book, feel that your own self esteem is low but not low enough that you need to see a therapist, go out and get yourself some good positive thinking books and tapes.

Have you ever said to yourself, over and over again 'I like

myself. I like myself.' Try it, feel the feeling when you say these words. Do you feel uncomfortable? Do you feel silly? Is it that you feel something will go wrong if you tell yourself that you like yourself – don't get too happy? What we fail to realise is that our self esteem is within our own heads. We listen so much to what others tell us about ourselves that we don't realise they may be covering up their own unhappiness by bringing us, and other people, down in order to make them feel good.

If you need to help yourself just say that sentence 'I like myself.' Say it over and over again.

There are positive thinking courses available. There are weekend 'inner child' courses or self esteem courses. All are available if only you look. These courses are designed to help you look at the good points about yourself. We never look at the good points. Instead we feel only the strong feelings we get over points we don't like about ourselves. Have you ever laughed at these 'bad' points? Have you ever been able to smile and say 'Well look at my strengths instead'? We all feel that the things we can't do are our weakness. Have you ever thought of turning these weaknesses into strengths by being able to laugh at yourself? The more you are able to laugh and feel at ease with the things you feel you are not good at, then the sooner you begin to be this person you have always wanted to be. The person who feels at ease with themself. The person we look at who is so laid back and relaxed. The person we were trying to be all those years ago. You don't need to be good at everything. Just look and remember all the things you ***are*** good at.

How do we define success? We tend to think it is a big car, big house, money in the bank, successful business. But is that really true? You can have all of these and still have low self esteem. If you believe in yourself you will have peace of mind. To believe in yourself you must be relaxed, at ease with yourself and with who you are, not who you think you ought to be. If you have peace of mind your self esteem will begin to grow because you realise that the secret of success is feeling at ease with yourself – waking up in the morning and feeling really well. If you feel well and if you feel good about yourself you can go out into the world and achieve the house and the car and the bank balance. Self esteem does not come easily to anyone. Self esteem is something that has to be worked at each and every day by telling yourself how much you like yourself.

3.3 Positive Mental Attitude

If we're really unhappy in our life we need to look at what it is that we're unhappy about. How many others do we blame in our life? How many other people are causing our problems? There is only one person responsible for your problems – you!

You can change your life no matter how impossible a task you think it might be. But firstly you need to accept responsibility for it. You must stop blaming others. If you are in a situation you feel you cannot escape, then the thing to do is change your attitude towards it and in doing so you will build up your belief in yourself. If you are unhappy with a person or a situation, you don't have to actually change ***them***. Instead you need to be able to change your own attitude towards yourself. People treat us as they see us and we treat other people as we see them.

If, for example, you are stuck in an unhappy marriage with children to provide for. You can't simply go out and make radical changes to your lifestyle. You can find yourself some more books like this one. Start working quietly on your own to raise your self esteem. Notice that you start feeling changes happening from within. As those changes happen inside we begin to deal with people and to come across to people in a different way. They start to treat us differently. They won't know what the change is but they can see something indefinable. People may say to you 'There's something different about you today, but I can't quite put my finger on it.'. That's exactly the reaction you're looking for. We don't want to suddenly change into an aggressive individual who's no longer willing to put up with anyone or anything. If you were to walk out of the marriage now it may be that you would have to leave your children behind. That's not easy. So start working on yourself instead. Start feeling different within yourself. Start treating people differently. Feel differently towards them. As that happens start making affirmations. 'I like myself. I like myself.' If you need a job, tell yourself that 'New and interesting work flows freely to me in abundance.' 'A highly paid and interesting job flows freely to me in abundance.' 'A highly paid job that is suitable to school hours flows freely to me in abundance.'

Make those affirmations. Watch them happen.

By thinking negative thoughts we are affirming for things we don't want. Affirm for everything you do want. Make those affirmations. Make them fun affirmations. All affirmations work. We make negative affirmations to ourselves every single day affirming our low self esteem. We do nothing about the problems in hand or about changing them, we only affirm to keep them and of how to keep them. Until now we may not have been aware that this is what we are doing. People say that they can't get their mind to stop working, that it goes in every direction giving them fearful thoughts and fearful feelings. Yes this does happen. I have felt this too. How do we stop these thoughts? How do we stop these feelings? We can't stop them immediately. What we can do is start today by making one affirmation 'I feel so healthy. I feel so happy.'

Make your list of affirmations. Keep it simple. Even for the fraction of a second it takes to say them you do begin to feel healthy, you do begin to feel happy. Your body reacts in this way to your thought processes. We have natural hormones within us – natural chemicals called endorphins. Endorphins that reduce pain, chemicals that make us feel happy. So if you expect to have negative feelings every day, you give yourself negative affirmations every day and give yourself these thoughts and feelings every day. So reverse them. It sounds so simple but, believe me, this is how you raise your self esteem, how you give yourself positive thoughts and feelings, how you change your life. Tell yourself that you are going to make these affirmations, whether it's while you have your shower in the morning or when you are lying in bed before you get up. What a good way to start off your day! How do we normally start our day? We start by giving ourselves so many negative affirmations. 'Oh no, I feel so awful this morning.' 'It's so cold this morning.' 'I've never been a morning person.' 'I've got to get up and feed the cat/the children.' 'I've got to get up and queue for the bus.' 'I hate this job.' You look forward to the weekend, but for what? Have you ever thought about how you feel on a Friday when you finish work? You actually feel for a short time a surge of positive energy at the prospect of the weekend ahead. Why not start giving yourself that surge every day. Tell yourself that you do feel happy, that you do feel healthy. In fact tell yourself that you feel really wealthy. Wealth doesn't have to be in the form of money.

Sometimes though we do have to affirm for money. People feel bad about affirming for money. Don't. Money is not the root of all evil. It can only be evil if it is used in a very negative way. Affirm for a job that pays very well. Make yourself affirmations that suit you. Make them as if they have already happened. 'I am very healthy.' Not, 'Next week I will be very healthy.' or 'When I feel better I will be very healthy.' Make these affirmations very positive. Make them for something that ***you*** want, not for something other people want you to have. Affirmations are one of the most exciting things that can happen to you in your life. Affirm for what you want. Never think anything is impossible.

Affirmations are putting into words what you have always

wanted to be, what you have always wanted to do. They represent how you have always wanted to feel inside but have never known how to make it happen. By telling yourself how awful you feel every day you are compounding the problem. Your body is reacting to exactly what you are telling it that you feel. By changing these thoughts (and it isn't easy) into a positive affirmation, just to continue telling yourself something positive over and over again you can make your body react in a positive way and change your overall outlook on life.

Affirmations can work whether you are having a panic attack or whether you feel you don't have any confidence. Obviously the affirmations you use would be different in each case. For your self esteem you would tell yourself, 'I feel confident, I feel happy, I feel well.' You would continue with that until suddenly, just for a few seconds, you would start taking in these feelings. In feeling confident and happy and well a whole new world opens up for you. You begin to see and feel things that have always been there but you've never noticed. If you are having a panic attack the affirmation you would use is 'I feel calm, I feel calm and relaxed.' For that moment just hang on to the thought that will see you through the attack.

When affirmations don't work immediately people give them up, stop saying them. They forget that affirmations have to be worked at. Why is it that thinking negatively in our everyday life is so much easier than thinking positively? It is simply a habit. Yet we can get so many rewards out of thinking positively and none from thinking negatively. Or do we?

When we think negatively it sometimes has a secondary gain. It saves us from stepping forward in our life. It means that we don't have to change our life. It gives us a reason to blame everyone else, an excuse for not stepping forward in our life. If we happen to be in a life that we can't change, (and some situations do have to be tolerated, at least temporarily) then at least we can change our attitude towards it and help ourselves feel better. There's no excuse left for not changing our life. What are we going to do in our later years? Will we still be blaming others for our lot? We need to step forward and take these affirmations and use them in a very positive way.

Affirmations will change your life but will only change your life if you continue to use them. For your first affirmations you should try 'I like myself.' and 'I feel really healthy.' If you start to tell yourself that you like yourself you actually begin to see things about yourself that you like. If you tell yourself that you feel very fit and healthy you begin to see sports and activities that you would like to try. Even if it's just walking, things become more interesting to you as you walk. If you tell yourself you feel healthy you start to feel very healthy, you start to feel better within yourself. You will want to go out more, start doing things. If you tell yourself that you feel very successful 'Success flows freely to me in abundance.' and keep repeating these affirmations then they become reality. How will you know when this happens? Believe me the rewards will be so magnificent they will astound you. In fact the results of affirmations are so powerful you may be frightened to continue with them.

Some people ask what will happen if they do affirmations to hurt other people. The truth is they won't work. The reason being that the only person who can be affected by your affirmations is yourself. Bad affirmations will turn on you and you will become a bitter, angry and resentful person. You need to do positive affirmations to help yourself.

Affirmations first thing in the morning and last thing at night are particularly important because you are at your most susceptible and your mind is most receptive at these times.

All those years ago when you were a child your mind accepted that you were a 'bad' person when you were chastised by an adult. You accepted so readily because in childhood we have plenty of emotion. When there is emotion your subconscious mind will pick up on things and act out what it believes to be true. So when you say your affirmations, it is best done at a time when you are relaxed and feeling good. When you say your affirmations last thing at night tell yourself how good you will feel in the morning. 'When I awaken in the morning I feel so wonderful.' 'I feel so wonderful, relaxed and I'm looking forward to the day ahead.' Your subconscious mind picks this up and as you awaken in the morning your mind and your body feel good. What a wonderful thing, as you sleep at night, to look forward to the morning! And to think you were the person who claimed they were 'not a morning person'.

As you walk along or sit on the bus, or your, car put on a positive thinking tape and affirm your affirmations. As you are saying your affirmations to yourself make them fun. Make everything fun. Enjoy your life.

Chapter 4: The Effects of Anxiety on Our Lives

Anxiety is not a socially acceptable illness. The symptoms aren't normally visible and the cause is generally obscure to the casual observer. We live in a society where stress and 'nerves' are supposedly cured by giving yourself 'a good shake' or by 'a hard day's work'. It becomes a shameful secret, the hidden epidemic. Ironically, the very process of admitting to the problem and talking about the experience is the first step to recovery and is the most difficult to achieve because of the stigma attached. Lack of understanding by others plays a major part in the suffering. Even our closest friends and family give up after so long at trying their best to understand, bending over backwards to help, lending support and making allowances for us. When nothing seems to make a difference they shut off, leaving us feeling more isolated and abnormal.

4.1 Shame

When people are stressed, anxious or suffer the effects of a nervous breakdown, they are, or feel that they are, labelled by others. People assume at best, that they are hypochondriacs, or worse 'nutcases'. This attitude is very hurtful, especially to sufferers of nervous anxiety who are, by nature, very sensitive and caring individuals. You can never be bothered by nerves if you are not a very caring person. Looking out for others and neglecting yourself has helped get you into this state. Friends may decide to ignore you because they feel embarrassed, others may simply feel helpless. Society makes us feel shunned. We, however, feel that we must keep a stiff upper lip and maintain outward appearances. Our world becomes smaller and smaller because we become ashamed about more and more things. You keep the situation hidden, keeping secrets even from yourself. You deal with it in your own way until it all crashes in on you. You blame yourself more and more, feeling weaker and weaker, feeling disgusted with yourself. All this time you never realise that every human being must feel like this at some point in their life. But perhaps they manage to hide it better than you do. Whenever a traumatic situation crops up you manage to put a face on it for the sake of others and what they might think of you. You pretend to be alright. I played the pretend game for years, acting out more roles than Elizabeth Taylor. But no-one gave me an Oscar for those performances, however difficult and convincing they might have been. A few years ago I bought my own 'Oscar' to remind myself of how I had made it through that traumatic period in my life. It sits in my consulting room today to commemorate the actor I used to be.

We are our own worst enemy when it comes to feeling ashamed. We yearn for perfection. We feel we have to be perfect, nothing else is good enough. We believe people won't like us if we're not perfect. We make the pressure greater. We batter ourselves emotionally and feel the shame of having 'failed'.

4.2 Roles and Relationships

How many people in your life make you frightened? How many people do you know who give you that gut wrenching sensation just by speaking to them? How often do you try your hardest to avoid someone?

You'll notice the feeling, the sensation in the pit of your stomach is always the same – different person, different situation, but always the same terrible, terrible feelings.

You are a victim.

You have relinquished control of your life to other people.

As long as we carry on having these feelings we allow ourselves to be swept along by other people's influences. In every situation we play the victim's role and that means we don't need to make changes in our lives.

No confrontation.

No unpleasant home truths about ourselves and about our lives being drawn to the surface.

Victims, however, don't make for good partners, friends or workmates. Victims are depressing. They talk depressing subjects and think depressing thoughts. What they get in return is pity. Wouldn't it be much more rewarding to earn respect and admiration? You need to stop being a victim in life.

People don't like victims.

So why do we take on this particular role? What causes us to become a victim?

Take a look at your life, particularly at your childhood. If you've grown up within an unhappy marriage, with arguing parents, then you will have subconsciously taken on the role of parent to your parents – trying your childish best to make life more bearable for everyone, trying to make their marriage/relationship better for them.

Perhaps you felt like a failure when things didn't always work out for them in the way you had hoped. How many times have you thought to yourself 'Please God. Please God I'll do anything just to make things better. If you could make things better for me I'll change. I'll change my life. I'll do anything.'

But bear in mind a child can never win in an adult world. Yet, you destroy yourself for not being 'brave' for not making things work.

So we progress into adulthood, acting as parent to other people, shouldering their burdens 'rescuing' them from problem situations. Sometimes these will be impossible situations.

Whatever our situation in childhood we learn to create 'comfort zones' within our lives. These consist of familiar situations and personalities. Often when we choose a partner we choose a person so much like the father/mother who caused us so much unhappiness in our childhood. This is not entirely coincidental. Such a person, believe it or not, falls within these comfort zones, representing what we 'know' and this gives us a sense of security. In childhood we grew accustomed to living in an unhappy marriage and that's where we feel comfortable. We know how to handle it. We know how to handle the people within it. We know how to feel like a failure.

Because of our childhood we don't know how to handle the person who will be true to us, the person who can really make us happy. You go out of your way to make your partner's life hell to convince them and to convince yourself that they will have an affair, that they are cheating on you.

The reason for this is the fact that you never saw your parents' relationship working, you've never seen a happy ending, you've never seen an end to the long and sad road they appeared to be treading.

The most frustrating thing about parents' relationship is that when you're young you think they will kill each other, when you're young you think they will leave each other, when you're young you think you will be abandoned by them in their unhappiness. What you don't realise is that you're listening to the words they're throwing at each other – not at you. But by listening to them they're actually getting the effect they want. The effect is felt through the children. Children are used as tools.

Men will often say to me 'Just give me back the girl I married'. How can I? The day that person got married was the day her life changed for good. That was the day she started to do the washing, the ironing, the housework, the full-time job and still try to keep herself looking and feeling attractive, have the children, cope with PMT this goes on and on. It's impossible to be the woman he married.

Under these circumstances it's little wonder a woman will start to doubt herself, to become frightened because she imagines her partner is looking at someone else. When this happens a woman can feel so belittled that she truly believes no other man would ever look at her and find her attractive. She begins to lose her sexual feelings, her sexual thoughts. She feels unattractive to her partner. In his own way the partner feels quite secure.

Then one day she may decide to attend a slimming class, an exercise class, an art class. She begins to take care of herself again. She goes back to work, the children are off her hands, beginning to take more responsibility for themselves and she has some time for herself.

Then the partner begins to feel insecure.

Sometimes he may be so insecure that he becomes ill. In becoming ill he starts the vicious circle off once more. His partner begins to take care of him. His demands begin to dominate once more. Her life becomes smaller and smaller. Once again he manages to get her to stop work and step back into his world, his small frightened world.

Eventually in relationships like this everyone says to themselves, 'If only I had done this' or 'I wish I had done that'.

They only have the 'If onlys' for the rest of their life, never realising that in each having confidence they could have become each other's best friend.

4.3 Anxiety and Sex

I have counselled in sex therapy for many years and, apart from physical trauma to either male or female body, the majority of sexual problems are the result of a breakdown in communications. Either partner can be too tired, or have problems, or perhaps they just cannot talk to each other.

When first I started studying sex therapy, many years ago, we gave books to our patients so that they could read and learn from them. Now we have sex therapy videos. (Not blue movies.)

These videos won't show you much that you probably don't already know about the mechanics of sex. They will teach you about communication, about how at ease you should feel with sex. If you are having a problem in your sex life, buy one of these videos. You will find advice on which to choose at marriage guidance centres or from your therapist. Sit down together and watch the tape.

Sex should be fun. If the fun has gone out of sex look at the rest of your life. Are you too tired or overworked? Are you trying to manage a job and manage the children? Are you pushing for promotion?

Look back to when you first met. All the thoughts you had about each other were very positive. The relationship was fun.

Remember the feelings you had back then about each other. Remember the feelings you had back then about yourself. It doesn't matter what age you are now, take yourself right back.

Close your eyes and in your imagination take yourself back. Feel those feelings, see yourself as you were back then. Imagine yourself back in your body as it was then. Imagine your partner as he was back then. Feel the positiveness you felt for each other, how life was a wonderful challenge. Feel all the good feelings that you had.

4.4 Making Changes

By now you're probably thinking 'But I've changed, we've both changed'. It's true everyone has changed, but think for one moment – just remember how you were.

Have you turned into a person who is bad tempered, who is fearful, who is aggressive or who has become very timid? Remember, people treat us as they see us. Which role do you play now – the parent, the child, the victim? Can you really lose out if you become that confident person once more?

You may think that you weren't particularly confident when you met. You may think that moving into the relationship was something that just happened, the next step in your life. If that was the situation for you then look at your life. Are you still reacting to situations as the frightened person you were back then? Have you grown stronger? Do you really want to find the real you?

Don't just step right out of a relationship and decide that you're leaving. Take your time, have counselling first. Decide what you really want. It can be a very lonely life out there. Sometimes it's possible to remain very good friends without feeling that you actually have to spend the rest of your life together.

We are all frightened people in our own way but we can learn to be confident. We can learn to like ourselves. We spend so much time disliking things about ourselves instead of concentrating on the things we do like and learning to laugh about the things we don't.

Which role do you play?

How does all of this insecurity and unhappiness affect your children?

How does it affect you and your partner?

You are entitled to happiness. Buddhists believe that we are all brought to earth into a life of purgatory, and that we should strive to turn each day into happiness and to give ourselves happiness.

Why is it we feel that life should be so harsh and so bad to us? Why is it that we're frightened to be too happy? Why is it that now we're frightened to be that hopeful person we were back then? The person who for a few weeks or a few months or a few years actually believed that life could be good, who actually believed that life could be exciting.

Become that person again for a second. Imagine it, feel it, see it through the eyes of that person, the real you. This is the person who no longer feels vulnerable or frightened, the person who feels loved, the person who feels at ease with themself, who looks at life as an exciting challenge.

As you become that person for a moment, let it become a few moments more – bring it into your everyday life. Start giving yourself that feeling each and every day. When you wake up in the morning give yourself that feeling just for a moment. Then a moment longer. You will start to see your life changing. You will start to treat your partner differently.

I'm not saying that you will fall in love all over again but, if nothing else, you may be able to separate amicably or make life better for those around you.

Often, people who are battered wives or battered husbands feel they get more out of the situation that has become such a large part of their lives. They actually feel they are important and that this is worth the abuse they are suffering. Neighbours enquire after them, invite them for coffee and a chat. They become known to the local police and have an on-going relationship with doctors and nurses at their local surgery. Would they get all this attention if the circumstances changed, if they gave up this role?

If this is happening to you, if you have become a victim, take another honest look at the situation. Perhaps, truthfully you are the powerful one in the relationship. You could change your life if you really wanted. There are refuges and there are people willing to help.

But is there a small part of you that says 'Yes, I could go but at least I know what to expect in my life at the moment. Nothing. So I can't be disappointed and I do have some small piece of security where I am. My family and friends give me sympathy.'

But, surely you would prefer to have admiration than sympathy? Your own admiration. Eventually people's sympathy will run out. They're going to realise that you could remove yourself from the situation, help yourself a little. So, think again if you are in a victim's role in any part of your life. You are an adult now, you can change.

If you are a young adult reading this book then you are obviously old enough to appreciate what is being said. There are organisations that will help you. In the past few years there has been magnificent progress in the setting up of organisations and help-lines to help people just like you. People can get help, children can get help.

Most importantly they can receive counselling. Counselling to help stop those guilty thoughts and feelings and stop the emotional blackmail creeping in. Emotional blackmail that is used by parents, by friends, by partners. Emotional blackmail is very destructive. When it is used on us we begin to learn how to use it on others. We then make those people our victims and the vicious spiral begins again.

4.5 Stress Drinking

Are you worried about how much you drink?

The first drink relaxes you – how often have you heard 'I needed that!', the second is nice, the third turns you into the confident, happy-go-lucky person with no problems that you so desperately want to be.

- But, do you stop there?
- Or, do you only feel well when you are having a drink?
- Do you drink when you are lonely, or when you have problems?

- Do you drink and dream of all the wonderful things you would like to do but never seem to feel well enough to get up and attempt?

If you have a problem with alcohol you may start to hide from people, feel your nerves are getting the better of you and go along to your doctor thinking you are physically ill. To get you through, you must first realise you need to face your fears instead of depending on something to make them more comfortable. You will have to face them eventually and wouldn't it be nice to enjoy a drink and stop when you want, instead of feeling that you need one to help you cope?. Drinking does not resolve your problems – it gives you some more! Remember though, even the best controlled drinkers do sometimes get drunk. So don't tear yourself to shreds if occasionally you have one too many.

The problem with a hangover is that it is only one third physical. The other two thirds of the agony is guilt. You torture yourself about what you said or did. You may feel that it is alright for someone else to say or do these things but you shouldn't. You might panic. You tense up so much that you feel a tightness in your chest and throat, pins and needles in your arms. You wake early in the morning and torture yourself into such a state that you cannot get back to sleep. You find yourself in such a state that you think another drink would calm you down. By now you are convinced that you are halfway to becoming an alcoholic. But stop and think for a minute. All the alcohol you consumed will have caused your blood sugar levels to drop. Eat something with protein instead, because if you have one drink you will probably have three and you're right back where you started.

Don't terrorise yourself by saying 'Oh God, look what will happen to me if I don't cut down.' say 'Well look what I can have if I do cut down. I'll change my lifestyle and do all the things I imagined I'd do when I was drinking.' Believe it or not, once you start to make your life more interesting, alcohol will not be such an important part of it. You will gather confidence, only this time it will be you and not the drink that wants to get out there and live life to the full. You must not depend on something other than yourself to get you through, otherwise you will not become tolerant to stress and stressful situations. You can only gain by facing up to things and helping yourself.

4.6 Pain

Many people live in their past even if they don't have problems. But people who are depressed will always want to talk about the past. They wallow in their own memories, thinking about the things they haven't achieved in their life. They recall the things people have done to them in the past and before long they're one of life's victims. They act out the victim's role and suffer all the unhappiness of the person who no longer takes control of their life.

When we are unhappy we suffer an emotional pain which can often lead to actual physical pain directed at a specific area of our body. Sometimes this can be a feeling of tightness in the chest and a pain in the heart. Is this the pain of too much emotion? Are we holding everything back so that our emotions become trapped within us and cause the hurt that we feel? Do we feel the pain in our back from carrying the burdens of so many people? Do our legs and feet hurt because we are afraid to step forward in life? If our teeth seem painful is it because we are holding words in, gritting our teeth to hold back what we feel, what we want to say but don't? Tension headaches can be everything coming to a head but we don't know what to do about it – a situation where it's time to let go or face up to it.

When we feel these pains the muscles around the painful area will tighten up to protect it and causes a secondary pain. Not every illness is caused by stress, but pain and feeling poorly can cause more stress. So, for pain to heal we must relax deeply enough to allow ourselves to recover.

Pain causes fear and fear is our only enemy. We become childlike when in pain. We think we're being paid back for being too happy, too smart. No-one is happy about being frightened or fearful because fear gives us the dreaded feeling in the pit of our stomach, the horrible adrenalin. Yet if only we stop for a moment and ask ourselves, 'What really frightens us? The answer is fear itself. Fear causes us pain, anxiety, high blood pressure, depression.

Have you noticed that when you're in pain and you are distracted by something you enjoy doing, the pain disappears? Have you thought about how many of the constant pains we suffer we actually bring on ourselves? By simply dwelling on a situation, thinking 'what if...' yet doing nothing about the problem, we may cause ourselves the pain and the distress and the knowledge that the fear has taken control.

Next time you are in pain ask yourself what it is that you fear. Often the answer will be change. People tend to deal with changes in their lives as being a fearful situation not as the challenges they so rightly are. If we deal with it as a challenge we can be flexible in how we choose to deal with it. We can change our mind. If you set out along a particular path then realise that this is not the right thing for you to do, then change your mind and do something different. No big deal. It doesn't matter what others might think. You haven't made a mistake. You've changed your mind and you're perfectly entitled to do so. Hopefully by now you realise that if others feel the need to criticise anything you do, they have the problem, not you. People need to criticise others to make themselves feel better because their self esteem is so low. If you judge and ridicule others ask yourself why. Who has judged and ridiculed you? Take time out to realise that it is not always the person on the receiving end of criticism who has failed. More often it is those who choose to criticise others.

4.7 *Analysing Why You're Analysing*

Why should you think about analysing your problems? If you analyse why you're analysing, your head will be spinning round and round, your mind in turmoil. We spend so much time negatively analysing our lives – why we've done this wrong, why we've done that wrong, why this is happening to us, why that's happening to us, why we should blame our childhood, why we can blame our partner, why we can blame the children. But nobody can make you happy except yourself. Whatever our problems, if we think about them in this way, even winning the lottery wouldn't change our lives. You might be happy for a while but gradually the discomfort would return. The way you react to certain situations won't have changed.

What you really have to do is decide that if you're going to analyse yourself you must do it positively. One of the most positive things you can do for yourself is get yourself into therapy. Having therapy can be a bit like taking driving lessons. Just as you need to find an instructor whose methods work for you, you must find a therapist who suits your needs and who makes you feel comfortable. It can be money well spent. If you can't afford to get into therapy, there are free counselling services available. Alternatively, there are self-help groups or perhaps telephone counselling services. There are also many voluntary services around the country who may be willing to offer counselling services free in exchange for some voluntary work. The Samaritans for instance, don't want anyone offering advice to people with problems if they've never experienced problems themselves. The Samaritans, Women's Aid etc., may offer to train you in counselling techniques, and in doing this type of training you will be getting help for yourself. Don't do this for all the wrong reasons, thinking you can get a free ride. These are very worthwhile organisations and often the people they have helped feel they would like to pay back some of the understanding by becoming counsellors to other people. There will be something for you somewhere in your area. Keep looking. Try your local clinic or health centre. If there really doesn't seem to be anything at all why not set up a self-help group? Get some self-help books from your bookshop or library. There are plenty around so stop making excuses.

We know now that we analyse everything in a very negative way. Why don't we use the energy to do something positive about our lives. It's the same energy. When you analyse negatively you are exhausted at the end of the day. When you analyse positively you give yourself hope, you give yourself dreams, you give yourself feelings. You always have something to forward plan, something to open your eyes and think about in the morning and to look forward to when you go to bed at night. You always have some aspiration, some daydream that you're going to turn into reality. You would be using the same energy you expend in negative thoughts and feelings.

One of the other reasons why we analyse negatively is our fear of success. We fear that if we do succeed, our circles of opportunity will become wider, creating more opportunities for us to fail and this makes life more threatening. There is no such thing as failure. The only failure is in not trying. We lose our ability to be flexible in our life and our ability to move forward, making life more interesting as we go. We like to stay within our safe circle where we can strive to be perfect and not fail. Even when we're perfect we're frightened of taking the next step because there's more opportunity, more chances to fail and we feel that we couldn't cope with this situation. But failure is in not trying. Success is going out there taking chances, making choices and making your life happy.

If you were to ask someone who is terminally ill what they would do if they knew they had six months more to live. They would probably tell you that they would do the things they'd always wanted to do and be the person they'd always wanted to be. They would no longer be the perfectionist. They'd go out and do everything they'd ever wanted because they would no longer fear failure. Why wait until it's too late for you. Put yourself in the frame of mind that if you did only have six months left to live what would you want to do with your time? What would you feel was important? What would be unimportant is what others might think of you. Most people you see or meet in your life are simply passing by. Why should they be important? They don't know you, don't know how you feel inside. Sometimes people go through a mid-life crisis and start to analyse their lives then. Suddenly, they have begun to feel old and so they have the excuse of age for not doing things for not getting on with their lives. Why wait till then? Go out there and give yourself some life experiences. You will become the most positive person you have ever known. You will feel positive. You will look positive. You will, quite literally, beam. Everyone will see the rays of energy you send out. Everyone will want to be with you. Everyone will feel the positiveness and hear the positiveness coming from you.

We analyse things in our life in a negative way because we are afraid of what others think of us. If you could actually imagine that you have everything you want in life. Imagine that there are no problems in your life. If you do have a problem right now imagine what your life would be like if it was no longer a problem. Think about it. There is no difference. It's how you feel about it at the time that makes the difference. Go forward as if your problems have been solved, as if your problems are no longer there. Feel the feeling of completeness, the feeling of positiveness you will experience if you imagine that you have dealt with your problem, that you have succeeded in resolving it. What you will notice when you experience these wonderful feelings is that other people's thoughts don't matter, the feeling is your own, it's private. Imagine then, if you dealt with your whole life feeling this positiveness. Imagine how different every day would be. Pretend can turn into reality and in the pretend it doesn't matter what other people think. Unknown to us they're actually thinking the same type of thoughts. They are afraid. They're worried about what we're thinking about them. Deep down we are really all the same insecure, unhappy people until we decide to change.

Go out into your life being that new positive person, playing that pretend game. Watch how people start reacting differently towards you. Notice that, in actual fact, you look at your life differently. You look at the problem you think you have and you deal with it differently. Now in your life, as in your imagination, you have the abilities to complete the problem, to take the problem into your control because you have decided to deal with it. Dealing with it gives you a new outlook which enables you to look at your life and analyse your problems with a different approach, a new positive attitude.

Chapter 5: The Road To Recovery

The purpose of this part of the book is to set you on the road to recovery. Use it like a map. Read it, learn it, always refer back to it. Keep it by you and trust in it.

More than anything else you may try, these few pages will pave the way to good health. By practising these exercises over and over, day by day, and building them into your life, you are laying the foundations for a happier, healthier future. When you read this, remember you are not alone on your journey. I am with you every step of the way. And remember also, that not so long ago, I trod this self-same path. It is long and arduous, but there is an end to it if you stick to the route. So don't give up. Use this book as your encouragement, as a friend and as a source of inspiration when the going gets tough. Which it will.

But first of all you should make an appointment to see your doctor.

Since the symptoms you may be suffering can be attributed to a physical cause it is important to seek medical reassurance before starting my programme of self-help. Your doctor may carry out a blood test to check your thyroid function, or perhaps a cardiograph to check the function of your heart. He or she may even prescribe anti-depressants, tranquillisers or beta-blockers.

You may find it hard to believe that there is no physical cause for your symptoms, that they are indeed induced by stress. This does not mean that they don't exist, that you are going mad. They do exist.

And you're not going mad!

It simply means that you have to find a different route to recovery.

5.1 Learning to Help Yourself

Once you have received the green light from your doctor, the next step is learning to relax – you have probably forgotten how. There are techniques to help, which you can practise almost anywhere, at any time and without anyone even realising. These techniques are a means of helping you to help yourself, to help you take control of tension – and of relaxation. Don't expect miracles straight away.

It may have taken years for your body to become as tense as you are now, so don't expect to 'magic' away the tension in one or two sessions. You must persevere.

When you first start using these methods you may not have

felt relaxed for so long that the feeling is alien to you. You may feel frightened as you start to feel good again and this may have the effect of making your body tense up again. It will take a while to trust yourself, to realise that it's alright to feel relaxed. Often when you first begin to relax you fear that something awful will happen to you. Don't feel too happy... because if you feel too happy something will happen to spoil it. How often have you said this to yourself?

The more you relax the more at ease you are with yourself. You learn to enjoy this natural feeling and you will start to take chances in life. Chances give choices.

If you practise one of these techniques every day and stick with it, you will soon realise that you can change your life. Recovery won't be easy. Indeed, learning to relax successfully may be the most difficult part of the entire process. Tension has become so much a part of your life that you have learnt to live with it. You have to learn to live without it, to turn it into something positive. This takes time and patience and practice and perseverance. Stick at it. This time you are going to take control of your life for once and for all.

5.2 The Tense and Relax Method

By learning to tense and relax parts of your body, pent-up

tightness and tension is released. This will alleviate the physical symptoms you are experiencing until, with time and practice, they eventually disappear.

For example, to ease tension headaches raise your shoulders up to your ears, tighten for a few seconds then slowly relax them. Do this twice. Press your head against a wall or against your pillow if you are lying down, hold for a few moments then release.

If you feel tightness in the chest, take a long breath in – not too quickly or deeply because you don't want to make yourself dizzy. Hold the breath for a few moments then release. Do this twice. The first time you will release the more superficial tension and the second time you reach the deeper tension.

Clench your fists and tighten your arms then relax. Do the same with your legs and even with your facial muscles. Lift your eyebrows, scrunch up your eyes, smile broadly even when you feel like crying. After each movement relax then do it a second time.

The more relaxed you are the more control you have over your life. As you try these exercises take your time and give your body time to adjust to the new behaviour patterns. Don't expect miracles overnight. The most important thing is to take it one step at a time.

Until you have practised these techniques and are confident that they are working for you it's best not to tackle difficult situations.

Choose a time of day when you are most calm and find a quiet place to practise. Make sure you can have 30 minutes without interruption. Take the phone off the hook. Before you go to bed is always a good time to practise because then you will also benefit from a good night's sleep. Be strict with yourself about finding the time to practise. It's always difficult after a hard day. When you're tired you can't see the point. Until you start to feel the benefits you must simply discipline yourself to practise.

- Don't expect to become fully relaxed overnight.
- Aim for gradual progress day by day.

Begin by seating yourself comfortably in an armchair, legs and arms uncrossed. Or, by lying down on the floor or on your bed. Breathe slowly and deeply. Close your eyes. Breathe slowly and deeply.

Make your body as relaxed as possible. Arms by your sides. Unclench your fists. Breathe slowly and deeply.

Concentrate on your right foot. Stretch your foot and point your toes. Now curl your toes. Scrunch them up and feel the tension in your foot, in your ankle and all the way up your leg.

hold for a few seconds then relax. Let everything go loose again. Feel how soft and floppy your muscles are, how heavy your leg is. Breathe slowly and deeply.

Do this once again with your right foot then repeat with the other foot. Breathe slowly and deeply all the time.

Keeping the rest of your body loose and relaxed clench your right hand. Notice the tension as it goes from your fingers, through your hand and wrist, and travels up your arm. Breathe slowly and deeply. Hold for a few seconds then relax. Do this once more then repeat with your left hand. Breathe slowly and deeply.

As you do each exercise try to follow the tension as it moves throughout your body. Pin-point all the different muscles as they become tense and notice how they feel when you let the tension go. Notice the heaviness. Notice how warm they feel. Let your breathing become slow and deep and regular after each exercise. Feel yourself beginning to relax.

Arch your back. Hold it. Feel the tension. Now relax. Breathe slowly and deeply.

Next pull your stomach in as tightly as you can. Hold it for a few seconds then slowly release the tension and let your stomach return to normal. Notice how good it feels. Repeat this several times.

Moving on up your body, hunch up your shoulders and feel the tension in your shoulders and in your neck, even in your chest and the top part of your arms. Notice how uncomfortable this feels and how your breathing is affected. Suddenly let go. Slump your shoulders as low as you possibly can. Let your arms become soft and heavy.

Now tense your neck by pressing your head gently against the back of the chair or against the floor – not too much. You'll notice how tense you become around your neck and jaw and how it spreads round to the back of your head and your shoulders. Release your head and let the muscles go. Breathe slowly and deeply.

Finally relax the muscles in your face. To do this scrunch your face up as much as you can. Start by creasing your forehead and frowning. Close your eyes very tight and clench your jaw. Squeeze your lips together and push your tongue against the roof of your mouth. Feel the tension. Then suddenly relax. Notice how you feel when everything returns to normal. Breathe slowly and deeply.

You should now be feeling very calm and much more relaxed. End your session quietly by sitting for a few more minutes breathing slowly and deeply.

It often helps to speak the exercises into a tape recorder then play it back as you practise.

5.3 Self-Hypnosis

Self-induced hypnosis is one of the most effective relaxation techniques available. As you become relaxed through self-hypnosis all the natural tranquillizers in your body will come to the surface helping you to feel calm more often.

Settle yourself in a chair or lie down somewhere comfortable. Close your eyes and begin to talk in to yourself (not out loud) counting from forty back to zero. Each time you breathe out count down another number. Should your mind wander as you descend through the numbers simply bring it back to any number and carry on from there. Don't worry if you forget which number you were at, any number will do. If you find that you keep going back to the same number, go to the one beneath it and carry on. When you reach zero simply go back to forty and start counting down again. Do this as often as you like. Don't be surprised if you feel that it isn't working at first. Keep at it. Quite suddenly your body will seem to heave a sigh of relief and slide itself down into a state of self-hypnosis. You will feel wonderfully relaxed and at ease.

By concentrating your mind you are not allowing it to wander to problems and worries. As you practise this technique it will enable you to sleep more soundly.

Brian

Brian hated interviews.

He applied for a new job, a good position with a large company, but began to panic every time he thought of himself sitting there before a panel of 'judges'.

Part of Brian's problem was caused by his lying in bed at night thinking of all the things that could go wrong at the interview. He was still tired in the morning.

I began treatment by giving Brian a hypnosis tape to help him relax. He played this at night in bed and fell into a deep sleep. He woke in the morning feeling rested. I then taught him to breathe in, hold each set of his muscles to the count of eight then breathe out, let go and relax. This way he became aware of any area in which he was inadvertently still holding on to any tension.

Now that he was able to relax I taught him self-hypnosis which would help him take control of his anxiety and teach him to slow down his breathing thus reducing the risk of a panic attack.

On talking with Brian it became clear that he had never really expected to get as far as the interview stage. He had applied previously for several jobs and had always been turned down. He was unhappy in his current job and so his self esteem was low.

In analysis we looked at the 'panel of judges' and Brian realised that he associated these people with everyone he had ever imagined was a threat to him. He believed that they would be able to see all the wrong he had ever done in his life. Brian realised that this was his reaction to anyone whom he felt held a position of authority. I told him to imagine them as children. Immediately his facial muscles relaxed. I then told him to imagine he was in charge of them. He realised that he felt good and that they were no longer a threat. I instructed him to feel a quiet confidence building within himself and to feel the wonderful feeling of well-being that accompanied it. When Brian opened his eyes he was smiling. He was aware that he could now perform the same 'trick' with anyone else he felt was 'better' than him or who posed a 'threat'.

Brian called to let me know that he was successful with his interview and was offered the job. He still calls occasionally just to keep in touch. His 'technique' for interviews has stood him well. He has moved on since then, climbing the ladder of success, relaxing his way to the top. He teaches some of his staff the simple methods of self-hypnosis and relaxation and passes on the tape to anyone he thinks might benefit from using it. Brian also teaches his staff interview skills and adds his 'trick' of seeing anyone who might be a threat as a child.

I find it most rewarding to know that after someone has been taught the techniques they need to improve their life that they are willing to take time to help others by passing on their newly acquired skills.

5.4 Practical Help

By practising these techniques daily you are preparing yourself for recovery. The first hurdle has been crossed. The journey back to good health has begun.

Set aside time each day to practise. Bedtime I find is best. And remember, the more often you practise the more relaxed you will become. When you are relaxed you are in control. When you are completely in control there is nothing to fear. When you have nothing to fear there is no need to panic.

To help with relaxation you should acquire a good relaxation or hypnosis tape. By 'good' I mean one which works for you. So try a few until you find the one you prefer. An enlightened GP may be able to supply you with a tape or try your local library or Health Shop. Good bookshops and record stores are also worth a visit. If you decide to visit a therapist he/she will make a personal tape to suit your needs.

Tapes generally fall into two categories. One covering the 'tense and relax' type exercises is especially good for tension headaches. The second type is a visual relaxation or hypnosis tape where your mind does the work, not your body. These tapes take you to a very tranquil place in your mind where you can totally relax. They will make you aware of your senses – hearing, smelling, touching, feeling. The place you will visit may be a beautiful beach or a favourite place in the country.

Should your chosen spot be the seaside, imagine you are standing looking out to sea. As each wave rolls in, feel waves of relaxation rolling all the way down through your body, feel the damp sand beneath your toes and the warm water lapping over your feet.

If you prefer the countryside, enjoy the exhilarating sense of freedom you feel as you are at one with nature. Think of a beautiful waterfall and imagine yourself standing under it with the cool, clear water cascading through your hair as you feel vibrant, full of energy and positively tingling with health.

Some people like to imagine a magnificent white light moving down from the sky. It is a healing, re-vitalising light which focuses on the body and rests on your scalp, progressing through the body internally, re-energising your vital organs and cleansing as it goes. See it shooting out through your fingertips and out of the tips of your toes.

Use your imagination.

A hypnosis or relaxation tape will speak these words to you. Although we don't realise it, human beings respond very well to command, so by lying back, closing our eyes and taking time out to use a relaxation or hypnosis tape we will benefit enormously from a voice leading us to tranquillity.

Others prefer to make this journey alone. There are, after all, many different types of people and many preferences. There are also many types of tape available. Keep looking until you find the one that works for you.

Don't worry if you fall asleep and miss most of the tape. This just means that the tape has by-passed the conscious or questioning part of your mind. It means that the tape's message will sink in faster and more deeply to your sub-conscious mind, in to the part that totally protects and takes care of you. If your sub-conscious believes that something is good for you then it will accept these thoughts and feelings and the process of change from within will have begun.

John

John had lost his mother ten years before he came to see me. At the time of his mother's death John was in his late twenties, very happily married with two children of his own. Since then, however, he had become very unsettled. He felt constantly that something wasn't quite right, that his mother wasn't at peace, that she wasn't happy. These thoughts were with him day and night and affected every aspect of his life. John's father was still alive and John maintained a good relationship with him because he felt that his father was much more important to him now. In fact, John had a great fear of losing him.

On the day that John's mother died he had been called to the scene and had tried to resuscitate her. He felt helpless, there was nothing he could do. His mother was actually dead before John had arrived so there was no need for him to feel he had failed her. Nevertheless John felt he had to try something.

John's problem began when he realised that he had never said farewell to his mother. He had never gone to see her in the funeral parlour and now felt that perhaps he should have done. For some people this is the right thing to do. For others it may be totally wrong. I have spoken to people who have taken great comfort from seeing their loved ones at rest and I also know many people who prefer to live with the memories of the person as they were when they were alive. John took the advice of other people and never saw his mother after she died. For years he felt he had never said goodbye.

I did an exercise with John that I use with people who have lost someone dear to them. I told him to close his eyes and for a few moments breathe calmly and deeply and to feel himself sinking deeper and deeper into the couch. Then I told John to take himself to a place he used to enjoy going with his mother, even if it was a childhood memory. If you don't have a special place imagine the person in your living room or bedroom or in the garden. John decided that he would go to the seaside. As a child he had spent many happy family holidays there. John began walking along the beach. He was alone before I told him to look out of the corner of his eye and he would see his mother walking towards him. John's face lit up – he simply radiated happiness. John had seen his mother just as she was back then. She was alive and well. He hugged her. He touched her skin and stroked her hair. He was able to tell her all the things he would have told her had he known that she was about to die.

Often there are disagreements in families, harsh words spoken to someone who has since died. You concentrate on these, think about them and torture yourself. By bringing her into his mind's eye John was able to tell his mother all his doubts and his fears and he realised also that this was something he could do at any time. He just has to sit down, close his eyes and take himself off to his favourite place where he and his mother can be alone together. He can go anytime he wishes, to seek advice, tell her his loving thoughts and feelings, share his hurt. He knows now that he need never be separated from his mother again.

Most people worry that, when someone dies, they will never see them again. They wonder why that person is never in their dreams. They think that person has gone for good and has shut them out. In actual fact it is the tension in you that prevents that person from appearing in your thoughts and dreams – you are shutting them out. If you were to take a few moments just to close your eyes, just to allow yourself to relax and to go to a favourite place with this person in your mind's eye. Talk to that person, hold them in your arms and feel how wonderful it is. This is your private time together.

Now John is much more secure and is getting on with his life. The feeling that something was wrong has just disappeared. He walks around smiling and people ask what his secret is.

5.5 Positive Thinking

We can all change our lives by simply changing our attitude. Positive thinking is one of the most effective antidotes to stressful and unhappy lives. Positive thinking can raise our self esteem, focus our minds on solutions to our problems and generate a surge of positive energy. The way we talk and think about ourselves and others provides the blocks which build the kind of life we actually live. If, every day, we expect negative feelings then negative thoughts and actions will take over every aspect of our lives.

Negative thinking is a habit we can't afford.

Making positive affirmations is simply putting in words what you have always wanted to be, what you have always wanted to do, how you have always wanted to feel inside. By telling yourself something positive over and over again you begin to feel it, for a few seconds at first, then gradually you will begin to see and feel things you have never noticed before. A whole new world will open up for you.

Affirmations will change your life if you continue to use them. Your first affirmation should be, 'I like myself'. Your second should be, 'I feel really healthy'. By telling yourself that you like yourself, you will begin to notice things about yourself that you like. If you tell yourself how healthy and fit you feel, you will start to feel better about yourself, start taking an interest in things around you and before long your life will take on a whole new meaning.

The best time to say affirmations is first thing in the morning when you wake and last thing at night. I use affirmations all day long – when I'm doing housework, walking down the street, whenever there is a free moment. I do it simply because they make me feel so good. Morning and evening affirmations are particularly important. Because you are at your most susceptible, your mind will accept them more readily. Affirmations are particularly potent when you are relaxed and comfortable and are therefore ideal for use during relaxation tapes or while practising self-hypnosis.

Set down your affirmations, repeat them as often as you wish. As you say them, feel them, believe that they have already happened. Believe that you deserve them. You can use them to improve your health, personal relationships, career. For whatever you wish for yourself. You don't need to sit down and close your eyes. All you have to do is repeat them over and over and over again. Either take one at a time or read them like a rhyme. The choice is yours.

At first you will be sceptical but as time passes you will begin to believe in them because you can see that they become reality.

Here are the affirmations I use for myself, and have done for many years. Learn them off by heart or speak them into a tape recorder and play it over and over again every day. They will begin to work for you. Adapt them. Use whatever wishes you have for your life.

1. Wonderful, wonderful loving things happen for me in my life today.
2. Wonderful, wonderful powerful things will happen for me in my life today.
3. I have a wonderful, wonderful power within me and it grows and grows and grows.
4. I feel very happy and draw happy events and people towards me.
5. I feel very healthy and enjoy the feelings of freedom that this gives me.
6. I truly believe in myself and accept myself as I really am.
7. Money flows freely to me in abundance.

Mary

Life is an attitude of mind. Regardless how many tapes, techniques or relaxation methods you try, you won't get anywhere at all unless you change your outlook. If you don't learn to change the way you think of yourself and of other people you won't make any progress. No matter how hard you work at your self-hypnosis or relaxation exercises you end up right back where you started – thinking 'nothing works for me, nothing can make me better'. And, to an extent you are right. Only you can work at making yourself feel better. The change has to come from within. Some people try out every kind of therapist available to them just to prove that no-one can help. We call these people 'groupies'. We all know at least one – the eternal 'woe is me'. 'Why does everything happen to me? Why must I carry everyone else's burden?'

Why? – because they love it!

Mary was a 'groupie'. People avoided Mary when they saw her in the street. Most of the people who knew her had long since realised the response they would receive to a polite 'How are you today Mary?'. Mary liked an audience and wouldn't hesitate to list her aches and pains, ailments and problems. Mary liked someone who would listen, someone too polite to walk away. She would latch on to people force them to listen as she complained incessantly.

Her husband was embarrassed by Mary's behaviour. Her children could no longer have friends to stay because mum was always 'resting', recovering from her latest ailment, usually something she had read about or heard of that day.

People were sympathetic towards Mary's family but Mary herself was treated with scorn. Which suited Mary – ever the martyr.

Mary wasn't too disappointed when I didn't make a second appointment to see her. I was, after all, just one more in a long line of practitioners who were unable to help with her problems. When Mary left after her consultation she was smiling, satisfied. After all I had lived up to her expectations – she was still suffering – and could continue with her tales of woe.

I feel no guilt that I was unable to help Mary. I only have time to help people who want to help themselves.

Chapter 6: The Power of Imagination

6.1 Taking Control

When you have a problem or feel angry, depressed, inferior or vulnerable, stand still and close your eyes for a moment. Let your mind go blank, and think.

Who is it in my past life, my childhood, my school-days who always made me feel like this? You don't have to be in exactly the same situation now but if you keep reacting in the same way every time you experience these feelings then the situation will never change. Things will never get better, because you deal with the experience in exactly the same way each time.

Who made you feel like this?

While you have your eyes closed, take yourself back in time to some of the situations in your early life when you did feel like this. See yourself as that child or that young adult. See yourself as that frightened person. Now see yourself as you are today and imagine yourself as you are now but reliving that situation in your past. Go in and protect yourself. Protect that child. Protect that young adult. Put your arms around them.

Tell them you have come back to collect them. Tell them you have come back to take care of them. Tell them you're in charge of the situation now. Tell them they need never again feel lonely or vulnerable. Tell them they belong to you now and that you love them. You truly, truly love them.

As you put your arm around the child, draw him towards you, feel his skin against your cheek, cuddle him. Let him know that you're there to protect him.

Keeping your arm around the child, turn and face the situation. If your problem is with someone you feel you still can't face, pretend that you can. Pretend that you're very brave just for that moment. Pretend that you can actually cope with this situation and deal with the situation for that child and for yourself.

Take a look around the situation and think of some of the things that person has said to you.

Look at them carefully. See them as they really are. You'll notice as you do this that they become smaller and smaller. They don't seem to be nearly so tall. They don't seem quite so big and burly. They don't seem to be in charge any more. Deal with the situation in your mind and rescue the child.

That child was a victim.

But you are the parent now, the parent of that child. Blend

that child straight into your body. Feel them becoming a part of you. Now, before you open your eyes ask yourself what it feels like to have that child inside you, to feel that child there, to feel that it belongs. It's a part of you.

Do this with different situations in your life. Protect that child.

Unless we do, we will continue to be frightened for the rest of our life and we won't know why. It's because there are situations we still need to take care of. Unfinished business.

Joyce

Joyce and her husband were referred to me by her gynaecologist. They desperately wanted to have a baby but Joyce had been unable to conceive. There was no evidence of any physical problem and Joyce's doctor felt that tension might be the cause. He was right.

Joyce and I talked about her life when she came for her first appointment. It soon became clear that the couple's sex life was now public property. The fun loving couple who had enjoyed the closeness of making love felt that they were now the subject of everyone's attention. They were having to endure the questions from excited friends and family. 'Has anything happened yet?' was well meant but to Joyce and her husband it became a particularly hurtful enquiry. Checking ovulation times and 'doing it then' turned their sex life into quite a serious business instead of the spontaneous stress release that it used to be.

Joyce's husband Barry came along to the next appointment. When they both started to talk out their feelings to me and to one another, the flood gates opened. There was no stopping them. It began to occur to both of them that there was a gap forming in their communication with each other. They had always been completely honest with each other, told each other everything, shared their dreams for the future. Their vision of the life they would share always included children – a little boy for Barry to take to football matches, a little girl for Joyce to dress up and show off.

They both started to use the relaxation tape I recommended and straight away began to sleep better. Realising they hadn't been sharing their thoughts and feelings highlighted the tension that had built up between them. They had been strangers to each other for some time. Together we reached agreement that they would give up trying to conceive, put the issue of having a baby on the back boiler for a year and that they would make love when they both felt like it. Fun is a particularly effective emotional de-stresser.

Meantime I worked with Joyce in hypnosis analysis. When I asked the subconscious mind if I could speak directly to the fertility part of her mind Joyce felt her heart speed up. This indicated that the particular part of Joyce's subconscious that ruled her fertility was stimulated, excited, waiting to be heard.

I asked if there was a hidden agenda, if there was a purpose to Joyce not getting pregnant. Joyce's subconscious state replied 'yes'. I asked what that purpose could be and the response was 'protection'. Further questioning revealed an incident in Joyce's past that left her with a fear of cancer. Her inability to become pregnant was her subconscious means of protecting herself from cancer. I asked Joyce's subconscious to take us back into her past.

When Joyce was three years old she overheard a part of a conversation between her mother and an aunt who had just undergone surgery for cervical cancer. What Joyce heard was her mother ask her aunt if she thought that having children had contributed to her having contracted the disease. Joyce's three year old mind had stored its own particular adaptation of the information and now years later her subconscious mind was equating cervical cancer with having a child.

I asked Joyce's subconscious mind to allow her to remember and hear the rest of that conversation. Joyce saw and heard her aunt reply 'Having children has been the best thing that could have happened. The cancer was spotted during a routine ante-natal check. I was able to have the treatment straight away and because of the quick diagnosis the surgery has been successful. I've been given the all clear. I was very lucky.'

Joyce was shocked that she could not remember the incident at a conscious level yet it appeared to be having such a profound effect on her own life. The fertility part of her subconscious mind was trying to protect her by not allowing her to become pregnant.

After a few more sessions with me to check out other areas of her life Joyce was a much more relaxed person. She called me four months later to give me the news she was pregnant – with twins!

6.2 The Child Within

As an adult you can cope with most situations, you know how to take control. So, when under any circumstance you begin to feel frightened, it's not the adult within you that is frightened, it is the child within who feels the fear. And because we either don't know about the child within us, or perhaps we know but don't acknowledge that she's there, we would never think of looking inside ourselves and soothing that child, comforting that child, healing that child. What we must do is relax for a few minutes, count from forty to zero or just concentrate on our breathing for a short time. Then take yourself in your imagination to a place you went as a child or to somewhere you find particularly pleasant. Just let your subconscious mind lead you there. Let your imagination take you on a fantasy trip to somewhere calm and relaxing. At first you may find yourself alone. If the child within you is very frightened she will not be there to meet you. Imagine yourself by a pool. Look into that pool and see your reflection. Look for the child. She may be hiding. You may have to coax her to come out from her hiding place. When you see her ask what it is that's so frightening. Put your arms around her.

This can be quite an emotional experience. You see yourself as a child and if you were upset or hurt as a child then it will be difficult for you to bring it all up again. This exercise is also useful if you want to rid yourself of situations from your past that are upsetting. Just go back as the adult you are now, put your arms around the child that you were, look into the eyes of that child and ask what it is that frightens them. You may begin to feel empty or you may feel upset or nervous. You may find yourself unable to sleep. This is your subconscious mind telling you something. You must go in there, reach inside yourself and find out what your subconscious is trying to say.

When you see the child within, put your arm around her. Tell her that everything is going to be all right. Tell her you've come back to collect her. She need never feel afraid or vulnerable or alone again. Tell the child that from now on you will always be there for her, that you will always come back to collect her. Tell the child that you love her, that anyone who did not love her had a problem, she did nothing that would make her unlovable. If you love yourself, you can love other people. Love is a natural instinct. We're all born with the capability of loving each other. We can all love ourselves. It is others who start to criticise and find fault and then we find fault in ourselves. As children we learn to dislike ourselves. We start to look for perfection in ourselves and the child begins to suffer.

Now you should take that child and blend that child within you. Feel the warmth of the child within you. The child is safe. Take yourself to other situations and comfort the child. At the moment when you feel unwell, or when you feel frightened, go in and collect the child.

Out of the corner of your eye, see yourself as you really are. The true you. The person who is very tall, the person who is very relaxed, the person who is very happy, who is smiling, who is no longer vulnerable, who no longer feels unloved. In your own imagination lift yourself up off the ground and into the body of the real you. Look at life through those eyes, feeling that quiet confidence within, feeling that wonderful, wonderful feeling of well-being. Feel what it is like to be the real you, the person who is very sure of herself.

After you have done this exercise, you'll feel very refreshed. It may be emotional at first, when you first see the child within. But when you start to see the person you really are, the person you truly can be, that confident person, then you begin to feel good. You'll feel your confidence growing and it will give you energy.

Sally

Sally had been abused as a child. When she came to me as a young adult she was overweight and unhappy. This extra weight was her armour, her protection from the outside world. When Sally closed her eyes and took herself into self-hypnosis, I asked her to look for the thin Sally. She could not be found. We called her and still she would not appear. We searched around and suddenly Sally said she could see her. The thin version of Sally was hiding behind a large rock looking happy and contented. She was stuffing herself with sweets and chocolate.

The uncle who had abused her used to give the young Sally sweets to keep her quiet. Sally hated the young Sally who must have allowed the abuse to continue in order to get more sweets.

Sally as an adult continued the abuse on herself in a different way. She called herself 'fat' and 'slovenly' decided that she couldn't get a boyfriend because no-one would want to be seen with her when there were plenty of thin girls around. She thought being fat was the reason she had no friends, no job, no qualifications.

But if she became thin the excuse would be gone, she would have to step out there and learn to get by on her own, to go by her own intuition. She would have to learn how to trust and whom to trust. She had trusted her uncle and suffered terribly for that trust. Her family knew nothing of what had happened in her past and were generally unhelpful by constantly deriding her about her weight. So, Sally would continue to eat sweets until she felt fulfilled and comforted and the vicious circle continued.

As the weeks in therapy went on, Sally learned to love herself as a child. She collected the child from behind that rock and blended the child into herself to find a feeling of fulfilment that did not come from eating. It took some time for Sally to make her recovery because she had become accustomed to talking and thinking about herself in a negative manner. By doing this she had her excuses for the way she lived. She was able to say 'how can I go out into life and take chances looking and feeling like this?'

During her two years of therapy Sally suffered many set-backs. Set-backs, however, are not entirely negative. They may be disappointing and frustrating when you are trying so hard to make progress but a set-back will highlight another area of your life you need to look at. Sally had to learn to trust herself, to know when she was being unreasonable and to handle other people's limitations.

In her insecurity she would keep pushing people to the limit until they made promises or arrangements that they couldn't keep. Sally would feel let down.

In truth Sally was still telling herself' 'I knew it. I knew they would let me down. Who can I trust?' 'Stupid fool you've done it again, trusted someone else and they've let you down. When will you ever learn?'

Sally was giving her new friends impossible goals. As soon as she was made aware of this she once again looked inside for the scared Sally. She would find the frightened child and tell her she was safe. Sally would cuddle the child, wrap her arms around the child and blend the child straight into her body. Sally told the child that she was loved, that she was accepted unconditionally.

Each time Sally had a set-back there was a specific reason, some area of her life that needed specific attention. Bear in mind that although we cannot live in the past or change what has already occurred, we can change the way we look at it. Sally continues with her own therapy now.

Everyone should try this method of finding the part of you that is frightened. Speak to the child within. If we were to deal now with the situations from our childhood that caused us so much pain and fear they would not seem as threatening or as fearful as they did back then. So take yourself back into your subconscious. Go in as you are now and rescue yourself. Fight for yourself back then but as the adult you are now. See the situation as it truly was and not as you have always imagined it to be. Notice how different you feel now that you are in charge, now that you have taken control. See the other people in there, the threatening people. See them as children too. Remember you are the boss.

Tell the child within that you have kept a promise. A promise to come back and collect them. Blend that child straight into your body. Then feel how good it is to have yourself inside, safe, warm and complete.

Sally can do this for herself now any time she wishes. She doesn't need to eat to feel good about herself.

Sally is in control now.

Chapter 7: Getting Better

7.1 The Benefits of Physical Exercise

Physical exercise is one of the most important aspects of your recovery because it gets rid of all the excess adrenalin that builds up. The excess adrenalin that causes all the symptoms of your panic attack. The excess adrenalin that causes all those horrible feelings. So take a walk if you can or jog on the spot. Do sit ups – anything will do so long as you make your body work. When you are panicky your adrenalin levels are building up and you need to get rid of it. You may laugh at the thought of jogging up and down the aisles of the supermarket next time you start to feel panicky, but quite honestly if you don't get rid of the adrenalin you will never take control. The adrenalin is what makes us feel so unwell and is what really depletes our energy. So, jog on the spot, take a walk, get yourself an exercise bike and take control of your life.

When you can't sleep don't lie there fretting and worrying about the fact that you can't sleep. Get up and do something. The best cure for insomnia is to get up and do something physical.

- Wash the windows;
- clean the kitchen;

- paint the walls;
- read a book or newspaper.

Don't be tempted to sleep during the day and after two nights you'll be so exhausted it will be impossible for you not to sleep.

Natural or herbal remedies for insomnia should be treated with caution. They can have side effects, some of which could be quite serious. People often disregard the recommended dosage because they assume that something which is herbal must be harmless. This is not always the case. You must make sure that you are not causing yourself any harm. Always check with your doctor before starting any kind of treatment. Your doctor is there to help. Your doctor is human. Your doctor has been stressed too and will be very interested in your recovery. Doctors are not gods and you should look upon them as your equal. This can be difficult when your self-esteem is low and you feel yourself to be inferior to almost everyone. But your recovery must start somewhere. Build yourself up with your relaxation exercises. These are the basic building blocks of good health. Then work on your physical exercise. This is so important because it rids you of the horrible feelings that the adrenalin gives you. You want to turn the horrible adrenalin into happy adrenalin. Remember there is no physical difference between the feeling of fear and the feeling of excitement (rapid heart, butterflies in the stomach) except the way you think. This will happen if you work at it. Each time you do feel a bit panicky you realise that you are taking control little by little until you know that nothing in the world can touch you. The fear starts to turn to excitement and this gives you the energy. At the end of the day it's much better to feel exhausted from having had a pleasurable day than to be exhausted and drained by feeling bad.

7.2 How to Deal with a Panic Attack

If you do fear the onset of a panic attack. If you feel the start of those horrible feelings you must catch them early, put a stop to them before they take hold. You need to know that you are in control. No longer is your life controlled by panic attacks or by the fear of panic attacks. By carrying out your relaxation exercises, by making them a part of your life you will gradually take more and more control of your life. Then you need not fear the start of a panic attack at all.

When you do feel the sensation of a panic attack coming on, look around you. If there is any actual, immediate danger to react towards then do something about it. If there isn't any real threat, if you feel dizzy or under pressure or are finding it difficult to cope then remove yourself from the situation if at all possible. There may be times when this is not possible but not many. Even if you are in an important meeting you can always excuse yourself and go to the toilet. When you take yourself away from the situation you will feel less trapped which in itself will help you to see things differently. Your panic attack will take hold whenever you start to feel trapped. And no-one traps you but yourself.

Even on an aircraft you are not trapped. You can't step off the plane but you can step out of your seat. You can move up and down, you can walk around. You can do something about your attack. You can take control of the situation. Why not take earphones and your relaxation tapes with you? Do something to pass your time. Have you noticed that your panic attacks come when you're bored, when you have nothing to do? You now have all the tools available to enable you to take control of your panic attack. Do your 'counting from forty down to zero' exercise. Concentrate on your breathing, practise your tense and relax exercise. You can do something that you have never been able to do before – take control of the situation. Think outwardly instead of inwardly. Notice things going on around you rather than concentrating and holding on to how you physically feel inside.

If you panic on public transport simply get off the bus, get off the train. Even if you're in Timbuktu you can still get off. Nobody traps you but yourself. Fear is your only enemy. Fear is what's holding you back. We are our own prison officers. We hold the key to our own cell. So, remove yourself from the situation. Get up and move about. Sitting still is actually causing you problems. Sitting still means you can't get rid of the adrenalin. You must remove the build up of adrenalin by physical activity. It will also take your mind off thinking about yourself. It is common for people to wonder why it is that you can't stop thinking about yourself. People feel that you have a very selfish attitude to life. You do not. You are ill and it is a simple fact that your life has become out of control. So, start taking control now. Concentrate on your breathing, get up and move around. If it is totally and absolutely impossible for you to move around then do some of your tense and relax exercises. No-one will even notice and your muscles will use up the adrenalin that's racing around your body giving you the horrible feelings. Talk to yourself. Tell yourself it's O.K. You're going to take control of the situation. You won't allow yourself to be trapped. Be very positive. It may take a few attempts to get it right, but you will find that when you actually start dealing with the situation, you begin to take it in hand.

Then you can talk to your panic attack. Challenge it. Dare it. You need never again fear it.

I always refer to myself as a 'recovered' phobic. I never use the word 'cured' because I know that if I allow myself to get under too much pressure if I allow myself to get overworked or stressed then I know that my subconscious is going to stop me. I'll start to have panic attacks again and I'll know that's the signal to start easing off, to have more fun in my life. I need more free time. So, I'll close my consulting room door and take time out for me. This is one of the more positive reasons for stress. It acts as the voice in your mind saying 'What about me?' But 'me' is usually the last person you consider. There's no energy left at the end of the day. It's all been spent on others. You must try to set aside some time for yourself at the end of the day.

Normally you'll find that physical exercise works well because again it gets rid of any pent-up adrenalin that's lurking in your system. You may want to sit down at the end of a hard day with a drink in hand but this won't get rid of the tension. It might disguise it but it will still be there.

You must take control. You must take responsibility for your recovery. You must take the responsibility for changing your life. You can change your life. You may have given every excuse you can think of as to why your life can't change. This book gives you every reason why it can. There are no more excuses. If you read this book there is no going back. You have started on the road to recovery.

7.3 Planning Your Recovery

You should practise relaxation or hypnosis exercises at least once every day. It's always difficult to set aside the 20 minutes or so you need to do this when you have a busy schedule, but you must. One of the best times to do these exercises is when you go to bed. Then you will achieve a double benefit – you will become relaxed and you will also sleep better. Your body will soon get into the habit of relaxing and you will now recognise when your body tightens up that it is reacting to a situation. This is the point at which you need to apply some self-help therapy. You must stop and think about the situation. Ask yourself why you feel the way you do. Why do you react to this particular situation? Look at the situation objectively. Why does it upset you? Or, why does that person upset you?

What is it that you need to address, something that you're obviously not dealing with at the moment. What is it that frightens you? Or, who is it that frightens you? Happy situations never give rise to these feelings, only situations that frighten you. Is it someone in your life who used to make you feel like this when you were young and now you find that you keep getting these feelings? Are you in a situation where you know you ought to assert yourself but feel that you can't? If you can remain happy and calm about the situation you won't feel like this. If the situation makes you feel uptight and you get the horrible feelings, you must calm down. Do your relaxation exercises.

As you do your exercises talk quietly into yourself. Ask your subconscious mind what it is that's bothering you and what would make you feel differently about it. Think about altering how you feel. Look for positive things in the situation. Take time out and do your self-hypnosis exercises. Allow your subconscious mind to give you the answer. Trust in your subconscious. There's no point in just dwelling on the situation. We need to know what to do about it. There has to be an end result.

Take a look at the situation in your mind. Imagine that you can cope with it very well. Pretend in your own imagination.

- How would you deal with it?
- How would you feel if you could deal with it?
- What changes would you make?

Do this in your mind over and over again. Then go out

there and deal with the situation for real as if it has been fixed already.

If it's something that you must deal with very quickly then you must be very aware of your relaxation techniques. You must be able to turn to them very quickly and use them to your advantage. Which is why you should practise as often as you can then you can have them at your disposal when you need them.

It is the situations in your life that you are not dealing with that are causing you to panic. If you are calm and relaxed it is impossible to be angry and upset.

- What feelings are you having right now?
- What do these feelings mean to you?
- Are you getting mixed up with your emotions?
- What does anger mean to you?
- What does sadness mean to you?

Some people talk about having moods. Moods are when people are very quiet. What does that mean? Does it mean that by being quiet they are not communicating? Of course they are communicating. Being quiet is a language in itself. Being quiet suggests that people are not talking about things. It's the things we don't talk about that cause the problems. Do you have someone you can talk things over with? Do you need to confront things with someone you know, your partner for example? Running away won't help. Keep taking yourself into self-hypnosis and deal with things. See how much easier it becomes the more often you try. It will become quite real for you to have this fantasy situation taken care of in your mind. You don't feel quite so defenceless. You actually begin to feel a bit more in control. If you can't do this on your own, try to find a therapist to help you work it through. At least you have an end result even if it is only in your mind for a moment. But for that moment you will act differently while you imagine yourself taking care of the situation. Those moments begin to make your mind and body feel differently towards things and you begin to take control. If your mind and body refuse to take control you must ask yourself why.

Do you like not taking responsibility?

Do you like being able to blame other people?

7.4 Self-help Groups

Self-help Groups can be a wonderful source of support and encouragement. Your local library or the services section of your local newspaper will carry lists of groups in your area. Or enquire at your surgery.

Different people need, and want, different things from self-help groups. If there is more than one in your area, go along and try them. Find one that works for you. Contact the group organisers, speak to them, ask them about the group, about how it could help you to help yourself. Someone might visit you at home before you attend any meetings. Then when you do go along there will be at least one friendly face in the group. If you find it difficult to go on your own, take someone along – most groups will be quite happy with this arrangement.

A good self-help group makes you feel good. Most group meetings will be structured. Most will include a discussion about how everyone is feeling since the last meeting, improvements and achievements and new techniques to try. A good organiser will realise how difficult it can be to attend such a meeting and will appreciate the courage it takes to go along. For this reason many meetings will begin with a relaxation session to help everyone get maximum benefit from the group meeting.

A word of warning! Self-help group meetings should not be an excuse to moan, to feel sorry for yourself and try to enlist sympathy from other people. A good group will concentrate on the positive, provide encouragement and mutual support. A place where you learn to laugh again, where you can swap telephone numbers and make friends.

People come together in self-help groups from all walks of life. The thing they have in common is the suffering caused by panic attacks. The reasons behind the attacks may be different but the pain is the same. For this reason many lasting friendships are formed within these groups. You benefit greatly from the time spent away from your home, the sanctuary which may have become your prison. Self-help groups make your world wider. But remember, you are there to help yourself. Don't carry other people and their problems.

And always, always, always congratulate yourself for being brave. Every time you attend a self-help group session is a huge step forward. Learn to feel good about it and recognise the achievement you have just made.

7.5 Moving Forward

Once you have started on the road to recovery, you want to channel that recovery into moving forward in your life. Of course you should take all the help you can find at first, and yes, you should use all the self-help material that is available to you. But ultimately you want to get these under your own steam using nothing but good, strong, positive thinking. So use all the material in your recovery, but aim to develop your positive thinking skills. You must be careful not to wallow in the recovery phase. Don't start analysing your life, your thoughts, your feelings all the time or you will begin to live like this. You will be afraid to let it go. And if you do manage to let go, you will begin to analyse why you're letting go. You must move forward.

Even when you're working well with a good therapist, there's a time to part company. There's no harm in maintaining contact with your therapist for help or advice, but don't get stuck in the vicious circle of analysing and then analysing why you're analysing. Sometimes staying in therapy can seem like protection from our problems; a security blanket for some people. Don't use it as a crutch. Move on. Get better. Learn to be truly happy with your life. Use your experiences to change your life, to go forward in your life. Don't get stuck in depression. Don't dwell on analysis. Don't stay in therapy. Move forward and get back into life. Life is for living.

Agnes

Having a nervous breakdown is the best thing that has ever happened to me, for in making my recovery, I have created for myself a wonderful life. Now I go anywhere I wish to go, do anything I wish to do.

This wasn't always the way. Looking back to my school-days I was a very nervous child. I was a fearful child. But, I was also a very beautiful child, a child who had great feeling, who had great love. But also I was a child who could not cope with the outside world. Being a very caring and loving person meant I was easily hurt and my emotions easily exploited. But many years ago I decided that I wasn't going to change the person I was. Someone once told me that I loved too much. That's not possible. They might have a problem with loving other people but I don't. There is no shame in being a very loving and caring person.

If you have cause to read this book then you must be that loving and caring person because the situations and symptoms I have written about will only happen to someone with great depth of feeling. Uncaring people sail through life oblivious to the problems of others until something traumatic happens to them. Only a small proportion of people really care about others. We know who they are because invariably they suffer great anxiety and unhappiness because of it. Perhaps about one person in ten falls into this category. The fact that you are reading this book puts you up there with them, the ten percent of people who really do care. Don't try to change yourself. We can always get more out of life than the others because we tend to look around us. We look at the sky. We look at the clouds. We notice the colours of the flowers. We hear the birds singing. There can't be anything more wonderful in life than being able to appreciate what goes on around us in nature.

But you must also learn to love yourself as well as other people. Concentrate inwardly on the very positive side of your life. The past is past. You cannot change it. But you can see it differently, put it into perspective. Love yourself. If you love yourself and feel good, everything else in your world works out. It doesn't mean that negative things will never happen to you. It does mean that when negative things do happen you will be more able to deal with them.

I wish you all the luck and success in your recovery that I have had in mine. I hope to pass over to you what I have learned on my journey back to good health. I continue to learn, each and every day. I have met, and continue to meet, many interesting and loving people. Those people who are not like us, who are not loving and caring people, we can learn to deal with them, to put them in their place. They belong outside of our world now. As you travel on your journey you will find new areas of your life to explore, new places to go and new ways of dealing with things. Isn't it wonderful that you can now turn fear into excitement? Isn't it wonderful to get up in the morning and feel that it's going to be an exciting day?

To help on your journey to a more happy and fulfilling life here are some useful points to remember:

- If you ever regard anyone as a threat or bully, remember that a bully can only be a bully for as long as you are willing to remain a victim. See the bully as the child they really are. You will envisage them becoming smaller and smaller and you will imagine yourself becoming taller and taller.
- Imagine your brain to be like a sponge such that when you become really tense a hard shell forms over the surface. Nothing can get in and nothing can pass out. To relax yourself, imagine chipping away at the hard shell until it crumbles away leaving the soft sponge again, taking everything in and allowing everything to flow out. (Don't forget this is simply an exercise – your brain doesn't actually become harder as you become more tense and anxious.)
- Remember that people treat you as they see you and we treat other people as we see them. If we

imagine someone to be very angry or to be very loving then we treat them accordingly. Next time you are in company, consider how you are treating people. What about your partner, your children? How do you see them, how do you treat them? Do you have preconceived ideas of what you think they should be, and do you treat them according to your own ideas of how you think they should behave? Or do you accept them as they are?

- As you begin to recover from your illness, as you become more relaxed, you will begin to change from the inside. That change will come across to other people and they will start to treat you differently. Someone may comment that they've noticed something different about you, but perhaps they can't quite put a finger on what it is. You don't have to tell other people that you wish to be treated differently. You don't have to shout and argue to make your point. Just start changing from the inside out and treat people as you would like them to treat you.
- If you are in the company of depressed people

for too long, you too will begin to feel depressed. It is also true that if you are in the company of people who are happy then you will become happy and positive too. When you can, choose the type of company you keep. Be aware of the fact that the more positive you are and the more up-beat company you keep helps you become happier and healthier in your life. Life is an attitude of mind. If you feel very negative for long periods of time then your body will react accordingly – negative feelings, illnesses, viruses. You seem to pick up everything that's going around. So think positive thoughts, feel good feelings, be with positive people.

- We tend to act in our everyday life as though people can see all the wrongs we have done. In actual fact, you are the only person who knows the truth about your life. So, you've made mistakes. Nothing is unforgivable, but still every time you think of those mistakes you get that horrible feeling. You cannot change what has happened in the past. You can forgive yourself and know that you wouldn't do it again. Every moment that you give to those horrible feelings is another moment of your life wasted. Think of the good you can do for yourself and for others by changing those negative thoughts and feelings into positive thoughts and feelings.

- As you cultivate and practise your new positive approach to life, remember the benefits of positive affirmations. When you do affirmations phrase them as if they have already happened. There are no limitations to your affirmations. You can affirm for whatever you wish. Remember 'you can and somehow you will'. Decide on your goals. What is it that you really want from life. How often have we made affirmations for negative things, for something we don't want to happen? We do this so often in our daily lives we don't even recognise them as affirmations, they're just part of the way we live. Don't depend on others to make your affirmations work out. Make them personal. People ask me if affirmations work. They do. All you have to do is concentrate and never give up saying them.

Summary

We are all entitled to happiness in our lives but we must learn to make that happiness for ourselves, to be constructive in our approach to life and to overcome the difficulties we meet every day. We must learn to overcome the tension and anxiety that can cause us so much pain and misery. This book is your guide on the road to that happier, healthier life that we all desire but only too often feel that we can never attain. It focuses on our need to change from within, to take control of our lives and to exorcise the influences of our past which affect the way in which we deal with the issues in our life today. The writing of this book was inspired by my own personal experience and is therefore written with the real understanding of someone who has been there, who has felt the pain and despair that only those who have suffered can truly understand. It offers guidance and hope and is proof positive that there is an end to the suffering.

Anxiety is not a socially acceptable illness. The symptoms aren't normally visible and the cause is generally obscure to the casual observer. It becomes a shameful secret – the hidden epidemic. The feelings we have of shame and isolation only compound the anxiety. We batter ourselves emotionally and label ourselves failures. Every aspect of life is affected by this anxiety, our roles in life, our relationships with others. We relinquish control, swept along by other peoples' influences. We become one of life's victims.

It's true that we all have problems but some people appear to cope better than others. It is, in fact, our own reaction to a situation which can have such devastating impact on how we live our lives. The anxiety we feel can cause such emotional torment that we experience an overwhelming physical and mental reaction that channels all of our energies to internal conflict. The unpleasant and frightening symptoms of anxiety are simply caused by increased muscle tension but, left untreated a growing fear of the feelings brought on by these symptoms can quickly degenerate into phobias and panic attacks. Understanding and controlling these symptoms is the basis for our recovery.

Few of us realise that breathing can be controlled and improved upon and used every day to control our physical and mental well-being. Controlling breathing to slow down the heart rate is also the secret of proper relaxation and self-hypnosis (a gift we all possess but are not taught how to use). Often our anxieties are deep seated and to make our recovery complete we must search for the root of our problems and deal with them.

While we may strive to understand and control our symptoms, our recovery will not be complete until we have control of our lives. We must begin to understand the basis of our personality, to understand how other people have affected our emotional development and to understand how the impact of our background and upringing has affected us as adults. We must use our subconscious mind to exorcise the past, to prevent it from becoming an excuse for our problems and we must reach the child that is within us to resolve our emotional crises. We must learn to harness the power of our imagination, to go back into our past and to deal with the situations that are causing us so much trauma today. We must learn the benefits of positive thinking and how to make affirmations that will work towards making our lives happier and more fulfilled.

By taking on board the teachings of this book, by using it to guide you through the bad times towards new and exciting times in your life, and by accepting it as an integral part of your everyday routine, you will gradually lessen the tension, stop the anxiety and deal with the panic. Remember, however, that it is normal to be tense and anxious when faced with a stressful situation. You are not looking for a stress-free life. Your goal is to learn to deal successfully with the stress when it occurs. The road ahead will never be easy. Accept and acknowledge the set-backs and use them to learn about yourself and your problems, to give yourself the strength and determination to keep going. You will have succeeded when you can face each and every day with the knowledge that it will be happy, rewarding and fulfilling. This book has been written as a recovery reference to help you achieve your potential in life. Don't leave it in the bookcase or on the shelf. It is deliberately concise so that you can carry it with you. Reach for it when you need support and consider it your friend. Consider me your friend for I have taken the path you are taking now. I followed the road to recovery and I would urge you, through reading this book, to follow me to a better life.

Remind yourself of the basic steps to recovery.

1. See Your Doctor

Have your physical symptoms checked by your doctor. Anxiety and stress can present very real and terrifying physical symptoms which can cause very real pain and distress. Often it is hard to believe that such suffering is not the result of some underlying physical problem and you should seek medical reassurance that your symptoms are indeed induced by stress.

2. Acknowledge the Tension

Although stress has become a much publicised issue in recent years it is often regarded as the prerogative of those in powerful, high-flying jobs and relaxation techniques are the current trend in corporate fashion. This is simply not so. We all suffer from stress in its many and varied forms, and tension is something we build into our lives without even being aware of it. Relaxation must become your top priority before you can begin to recover from anxiety and panic attacks.

3. Learn to Relax

Practise relaxation each and every day. It is the most important advice I can offer and it is also the most difficult part of your recovery. Find the time each day to practise the tense-and-relax technique or self-hypnosis. Do it as often as you can but do aim for at least two sessions every day. Bedtime is one of the best times because it has the added bonus of promoting a good night's sleep. Find a relaxation tape that works for you. Take yourself to a tranquil place in your mind and become more aware of your senses – hearing, smelling, touching, feeling. Everyone is different and what works for someone else may not work for you. Keep trying until you find what works best for you personally.

4. Think Positively

We can all change our lives simply by changing our attitude. This is easy to say and easy to do but can be very difficult to believe. In actual fact positive thinking is one of the most effective antidotes to stress and unhappiness, but we can't bring ourselves to accept that our problems are not so large that they can't be overcome by something so simple. When we expect negative feelings then negative thoughts and actions begin to take over our lives. Negative thinking is simply a bad habit. Breaking that habit will take perseverance but it must be done. Learn to see the positive side of every situation and learn to appreciate the good things in your life. Count your blessings, they will always out-number your problems.

5. Make Affirmations

Making positive affirmations is simply putting in words what it is that you want from life. By telling yourself something positive over and over again you begin to feel it and gradually your life will open up and take on a whole new meaning. Set out your affirmations and say them throughout the day as often as you can. You don't need to sit down and close your eyes to say them. Build them into your life. Repeat them over and over. Say them as though you mean them. As time passes they will become reality.

6. Use Your Imagination

Often our suffering has its source somewhere in our past so far back and deep rooted that we are not even aware of the problem. We simply react now to certain situations which trigger the symptoms of our anxiety. Because we keep reacting in the same way when we experience these feelings things don't change and we can't move on. What is it that has caused these reactions? Close your eyes and ask your subconscious mind to contact that part of you or that situation which makes you most vulnerable. See yourself taking control of the situation. See it being corrected now as it should have been then. Use self-hypnosis. It will take you where you need to go.

7. *Accept the Child Within*

Adults have learned by experience to cope with most situations. So when you feel fear and anxiety it is the part of you that is still the child within who feels the fear. To deal effectively with these feelings you must acknowledge the existence of the child within. You must relax and let your subconscious mind lead you to a calm place where you must look for the child. When you find her you must soothe and comfort her for she is the part of you that is most vulnerable. Reach inside yourself and collect your inner child, love her and protect her. Give her confidence and make her safe. Through this you will begin to love yourself. When you love yourself you will look at life with confidence and a wonderful feeling of well-being.

8. Look After Your Health

Build yourself up with your relaxation exercises. These are the basic building blocks of good health. Then work on your physical exercise. This is important because it gets rid of excess adrenalin. The adrenalin that causes the physical symptoms of your panic. You must remove the build up of adrenalin by physical activity. Build exercise into your daily routine. If you are not physically fit and well you may be more prone to psychological or nervous problems. Good diet, exercise and sleep are all factors for a healthy mind as well as a healthy body. If you suffer from stress, your body needs all the help it can get, so look after it.

9. Commit Yourself

A programme of self-help therapy will fail simply because people expect miracles. When one session of relaxation doesn't bring instant relief you give up. When one recital of your affirmations doesn't give a result you assume they don't work. The tension has probably built up over many years and it will take some time to get rid of it. You will need some time to get used to feeling relaxed again. You must commit yourself wholeheartedly to the programme and this is the most difficult part. When you are feeling so fearful, so miserable and so unhappy you think there is no end to the suffering and the effort it takes to push yourself towards making that recovery is enormous. I know this from experience. But you must. There is no other way.The more often you practise your relaxation techniques the more relaxed you will become. When you are relaxed you are in control. When you are completely in control there is nothing to lose. When you have nothing to lose there is no need to panic.

10. You can do it!

You will do it!

Go for it!